THE UNSHACKLED MIND

THE UNSHACKLED MIND

HOW TO POSITIVELY COPE WITH RACISM AND BIGOTRY

ALMAS J. SAMI'

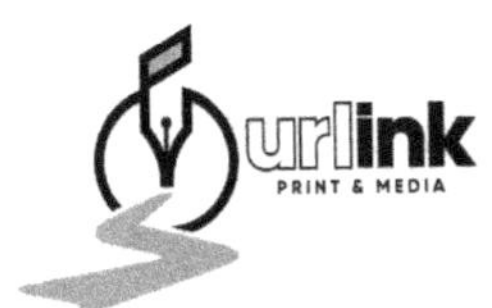

The Unshackled Mind

1603 Capitol Ave., Suite 310 Cheyenne, Wyoming USA 82001
1-888-980-6523 | admin@urlinkpublishing.com

URLink Print and Media is committed to excellence in the publishing industry.

Published in the United States of America

ISBN 978-1-64367-266-3 (Paperback)
ISBN 978-1-64367-265-6 (Digital)

Non-Fiction
13.02.19

I dedicate this book to Kai Sami' … my Wife,
soul mate, and bearer of my three wonderful children.
and also to my mother, George Ann Rogers.
Through the presence of these strong African women,
I am reminded that God is indeed good.
To my father, Almas Stevenson, Sr., now an ancestor.
a powerful and commanding Black man who did it his way;
bowing to no one.

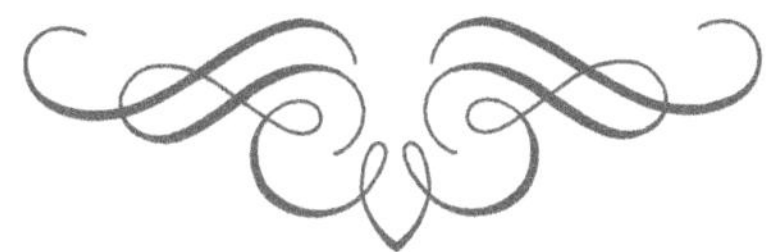

CONTENTS

Acknowledgments 9
A Note From The Author About The 3rd Edition 12
A Note From The Author About The 2nd Edition 13
Introduction 17

1. Farewell To Slavery 25
2. Roar With The Lions 44
3. Perceptions 51
4. Your Mind, Your Guidance System 60
5. Desire 71
6. Racism 78
7. Faith 94
8. Success 101
9. Myths . . . Breakin Barriers 107
10. Direction 114
11. Unshackled 124

Afterword: The Change Before The Name 129
Testimonials For The Unshackled Mind
Lecture & Book Series 145-151
Biography 153
Bibliography 155

ACKNOWLEDGMENTS

I respectfully bow before my God. May I find a way to consistently confine myself to the constraints, boundaries and limits of all that is good, natural and Godly. I also yield to my ancestors, near and ancient; all grand, noble and extraordinary. I would like to thank the many people, (both loved ones and enemies) for their contributions to this work. For no man nor woman in this realm stands alone and goes completely unaffected either positively or negatively by outward influences and circumstances. I am forever indebted to my father, Almas Stevenson Sr., and mother, George Ann Rogers for bringing me into this sphere of existence. They laid the psychological foundation needed to go beyond even my own expectations. My bold father taught me to stand alone, and my magnificent mother has always encouraged me to reach for the heavens. My off-spring, Sofi, Hakeem and Jamila, who have all contributed to the completion of this project. They motivate me, teach me and somehow find time to learn a few things from me as well. I am and will always be a proud Baba (father). My brothers, Mustafa and B.C. for their always grand show of support and encouragement. They have always taken care of little brother. To Dennis Smith and Vernon Cooper for being my very best friends. They are always in my corner eagerly waiting to assist me in any capacity. To Kai, Grace Naji and again Mustafa, for their careful editing and powerful critical review; they really stretched me to my outer limits. My librarian, Sue Heck for her kind and patient assistance.To Tom Martin, my first printer, mentor and friend, certainly providing proof that we *can* do business with each other and be met with successful ends! And last but certainly not least, a heart felt thanks to my wife, Kai, who stayed with me through more thick than thin over the past 47 years! There is not a single worth while endeavor, or notable accomplishment of ours that she is not directly responsible for. She is truly the most incredible person I have ever known, and I am constantly thanking my God for letting her share this life with me! And to my grand babies: Charles, Yamina, Aria, Chionesu and Lola. This is definitely my favorite crowd! Collectively, they inspire and move me to tears of joy often and redefine for me "what love looks like". I have infinitely more hope for human kind tomorrow because I know them personally. My Ancestors rejoice!

IF I COULD TOUCH

IF I COULD JUST TOUCH THE OTHER SIDE,
THE SPLENDOR OF COURAGE, THE
SATISFACTION OF WHOLENESS...

IF I COULD ONLY TOUCH THAT MAGIC THAT
FUSES MY INNER CONTEMPLA-
TIONS WITH OUTER REALITIES...

IF I COULD TOUCH TODAY, THE ETERNAL
NOW...

MY GOD, IF I COULD ONLY TOUCH MYSELF, I
COULD TOUCH ALL OF HUMANKIND!

Almas J. Sami'

A NOTE FROM THE AUTHOR ABOUT THE 3RD EDITION

I am submitting this Third Edition to "The Unshackled Mind How To Positively Cope With Racism And Bigotry".

Times are a changing it seems. Since the election of one President Barack H. Obama, we have witnessed a subsequent surge of racism and plain old fashioned bigotry. Of course we as African Americans and Blacks have always known that a certain amount of hatred was imbued just beneath the surface and more often than not chosen to be ignore.

A NOTE FROM THE AUTHOR ABOUT THE 2ND EDITION

I decided, for this second printing to address some of the concerns of readers who talk to me about this work. One brother said to me,"It's a good book, but its kinda short on instruction, ain't it? I mean, you don't tell us where to go, or what to do, ya know?" I can only smile, nod and pretend to understand. But the truth of the matter is that I didn't know what in the world the brother was talking about. So it occurred to me that he wanted a book that had THE answers. THE solutions. THE way. He was looking for a SAVIOR! Perhaps the second coming of Dr. Martin Luther King, Jr. or Minister Malik Shabazz (Malcolm X). I got the impression that he was disappointed with the work. Well, you too will be disappointed if you purchased this book with the intentions of being "saved" from your foolish inclinations, destructive habits and self-generated anguish. Please excuse my blunt manner, but I want you to know up front that YOU are responsible for your own life. You are destined to correct what character flaws need be banished. And you, my friend were given the power by your God to Unshackle your OWN mind! Do not expect this book, or any other book to free you from yourself. Only you can do that. It is not a jump starter for one who is not so inclined to seek to better themselves in mind, body and spirit. If however, you approach "The Unshackled Mind" with mental cleansing in mind, then you will be richly rewarded. For this book is intended to be utilized as a tool for those who are already at work on themselves! The overwhelming numbers of satisfied readers who I receive letters from give credence to the fact that most of us are interested in making our lives better. You are in for a treat if you purchased "The Unshackled Mind" with self improvement being your primary aim.

This work will take you for a pleasant ride down the side alleys and by ways of your thought processes. Some passages will make you rethink many of your positions about Africa, Africans, African Americans, Negros, Coloreds, Blacks and every other label that we are collectively "tagged" . You will rethink your positions on racism, racist and bigotry, and how they do or do not affect your life. You will also note that I have often used the term "African" in the place of "Black" throughout this edition. It is primarily because I consider myself an African with Choctaw blood. Notice that I did not say, "Black with Red blood. If I did refer to myself as Red, you would probably think there was something wrong with me. We Africans, the world over are the only humans who do not refer to ourselves with our place of origin prominently declared. It is not uncommon to see other people refer to their ancestor's place of origin when identifying themselves. Sly Stallone, Robert De Niro and John Travolta are shamelessly Italian. Thereby referring to themselves as Italian Americans. There are Irish Americans. Polish Americans. English Americans. French Americans.

There are even so-called mixed breeds or mulattos who refer to themselves as Irish and "Black" and the like. However, you seldom if ever hear anyone calling themselves Irish and African or Italian and African, etc. We avoid the label African like it was a death sentence! I am not against the term "Black" by any stretch of the imagination. But I know that my ancestors appreciate the fact that I pay tribute to the motherland by identifying myself as an African. Ultimately, you will discover that there is nothing new under the sun. For you in fact, already know everything you need to know to go where ever it is you seek to go in this life. You may not have all of the expertise yet; but you will learn *"how"* to get *"what"*... "where" to get "what" ... and "what" to get "where."

In other words, you either already have all of the answers or you have access to all of the answers. The Unshackled Mind will assist you in recognizing this truth. Good luck and hopefully we will meet in our travels. Do not hesitate to let me know what you think. I will listen. And if I do not understand what in the world you're talking about, I will still smile and nod — and consider you a cherished friend. (But remember; I do not instinctively know which portions of the book pertain to your particular situations and mindsets. For some reason, many people falsely believe that I can see right through them and pinpoint a malady or personal vice written about in the book. Nothing could be further from the truth. If you happen to identify with a certain portion of The Unshackled Mind, then that is between you and your concept of The Creator. All of the issues addressed in the book reflect my own past vices and maladies. I am simply sharing with you a portion of myself. We are all in this together. And that is why we identify so readily with certain passages, **and with one another.**) In the words of another very good friend of mine, Dr. William Harris, "It is never too late to address the need, whether realized or not, to do some serious *shackle shuckin*."

Enjoy the read, and make your life a good one. Unshackle your mind!

Brotherly,
Almas J. Sami'

INTRODUCTION

An **Unshackled Mind** is first and foremost a mind that has a *working understanding* of history! What do I mean by '*working understanding?*' It is simply an understanding of our past that takes the African or Black mind beyond our relatively brief history on this land. We have been in America for just a few hundred years... yet our existence in this world falls between 4,000,000—7,000,000 years! In other words, *collectively*, we know a very small percentage of our history! And most of *this* percentage is based on misinformation! No one expects the average person to be a history buff, however, a thorough historical overview would leave the *collective* with a calm and steady pride... a bond, critical insight and a glowing self love. This work looks back into our past, and pulls the reader closer to solutions to our *collective* problems of today. I believe the only way to address the concerns of today as well as tomorrow is by familiarizing ourselves *collectively* with the ancients.

The importance of history cannot be underestimated. The great historical mind, **John Henrik Clarke,** gave the most riveting explanation of the value of history when he said, **"History is a clock that people use to tell their political and cultural time of day. It is also a compass that people use to find themselves on the map of human**

geography. The role of history is to tell a people what they have been, and where they have been, what they are, and where they are. The most important role that history plays is that it has the function of telling a people where they still must go and what they still must be! History should tell a person who they are, where they came from, and what their potential is as a people!"

Without question, our *collective* minds have been shackled since our arrival to this land... as well as being shackled from arm to arm; leg to leg. In fact, the arm and leg shackles were not removed until the slave was well into the indoctrination or mind-shackling process. Once the mind was adequately shackled, the manacles were removed, and the newly formed slave was free only to do the masters bidding.

The American Heritage Student's Dictionary defines shackle as : **"1. A metal ring fastened or locked around the wrist or ankle, especially one of a pair that are chained together and used to confine or restrain a prisoner. 2. Anything that confines or restrains: the shackles of ignorance." It is definition #2 that this book will address. For it is up to us to correct the lies and misinformation about our past.**

In this late hour since our captivity, we are *collectively*, still languishing in the rear in the area of self-esteem and personal/racial pride. This will not change until we continuously seek to re-educate ourselves. It is our sole responsibility! No other race can do this for us. This realm of existence will surely remain psychologically painful for us until we remove the *shackles of ignorance* from our own minds. The agony of being African has been a burden that we have toted around for 400 years! The burden of pain will be lifted as we reacquaint ourselves with ourselves... distant past, recent past and present.

The color that our pre-slavery ancestors wore with an unbridled pride, has been a constant source of shame and self-hatred for modern Blacks. This was not something that just *happened* accidentally! We did not just wake up one day and decide that black skin was ugly, or big lips were unsightly, or kinky hair was "bad hair" or European names were superior.

No, we were decidedly sold a bill of goods. Our captors consciously sat out to shackle our minds so that we would hate ourselves, and love them ... so that ultimately, we would become better slaves. A knowledgeable slave was a dangerous person. A racially proud slave would be a handicap to the whole operation. Keep them ignorant of themselves. Feed them lies about themselves. Control their think- ing and they will make not only good slaves, but willing slaves!

Do you doubt me? In 1832 there was a White fellow by the name of Henry Berry who addressed the Virginia House of Delegates. He revealed much light on the plan to shackle the minds of Africans when he said; "We have as far as possible, closed every avenue by which light may enter the slaves' mind. If we could extinguish the capacity to see the light, our work would be complete; they would then be *on the level with the beast ...*" My purpose in presenting this work is not to preach, but rather to offer some of my own thoughts and observations on why I believe we are *collectively* functioning as a disjointed and disoriented family. Maybe you will see yourself in some of the pictures I paint. It is my wish that you will find this book thought-provoking as well as inspiring! If not moved to action, at least moved to "*think*," which is a requisite to action.

One may wonder why the first and second edition is subtitled, "An *Afrocentric* Approach to Self-Help;" given Molefi Asantes' anti-Arab/anti-Islamic proclamations in his past works. In his book, "Kemet, Afrocentricity and Knowledge," he defines Afrocentricity as *"groundedness which* allows the student of human culture investigating African phenomena to view the world from the standpoint of the African." I am in agreement. However, I have made a departure from Bro. Asantes' definition of what is and what is not deemed *"African phenomena."* I fall in line with Dr. Khalid Abdullah Tariq Al-Mansour and also the great 9th century historian 'Uthman 'Amr Ibn Bahr Al-Jahiz and therefore agree with their conclusions that there is a Black African presence in not only the foundations of Islam, but Arabic culture in general. We must investigate, if not embrace, African-Arabian culture if we yearn to embrace so-called "African History" in its entirety.

Yes, we must embrace other African belief systems and cultures... the Ashanti, Ghana, Songhai and Mali empires. Also, the intricate Dogon peoples, and the host of other systems that are reflective of our people. But how many of us today actively seek to embrace the teachings of the great Black preacher from India, Prince Sidhartha who today is affectionately known as; **The Buddha**, "the enlightened one"? Or what about the great Blacks who created China's first dynasty; the Shang dynasty over 3,000 years ago! Have we at all investigated the mighty ancient African Christians of Ethiopia? Our histories are too vast and encompassing for us to continue embracing only fragments of our past; and foolishly hold that these bits and pieces are in and of themselves complete.

Although I emphasize natural laws that govern all humans, this book is written by an African man, with African people in mind, thus, for the benefit of African people. For this I offer no apologies. But by the same token, I hold no malice in my heart toward other races. However, it has been my observation that we have too often given attention to the White tribes' attitudes and engagements and thereby have overlooked common sense directions that we should feel compelled to investigate on our own behalf and of our own volition. Quite simply, it is my belief that we will forever be held in "*psychological*" bondage until all people from **Alkebulan** ceases seeking White approval to think, to be, to act!

This notion is quite foreign to most Africans, for we are use to viewing the entire world through Eurocentric or White lenses. Hence, our people are afraid to seek truth as truth pertains to us. Even in this late hour, many of us will cling to European values and fight for those values to the very end — indeed, to the continued demise of us all! This is not to suggest that all European values are a detriment to people of color. However, we must recognize the fact that we are entangled in a system that teaches us that we contributed absolutely *nothing* to civilization prior to slavery! With this perspective, how can we not view ourselves as second rate humans? To view our world through Afrocentric lenses allows us, in fact, compels us to place our race among every other race as contributors to the world at large.

Ignorance of history entraps and enslaves a people and renders them functionally useless as a *collective*. The Japanese knew this at the end of World War II when the occupying American Government attempted to eliminate the teaching of Japanese history in all Japanese schools... the Japanese would have nothing to do with such a foolish notion! For they knew that the first generation of Japanese that grew up without the proper knowledge and understanding of their history would be a useless and spineless generation indeed! They knew that it would be impossible for their children and their children's children to unite, or function as a collective. Without a historical connection, they would fight, backbite and contrive to hold one another down. Distrust, envy and jealousy would be the order of the day. Does this sound familiar?

We African Americans not only do not know our history; we do not think there is a *need* for history! Hence we are mentally shackled and will remain as such until we touch base with a different concept of who we are now based upon who we once were! **WE MUST LEARN WHO WE ARE!!**

We must no longer use White perspectives and expectations as measuring sticks against the backdrop of our every thought and achievement. For instance, we teach in this country that Charles Drew was the first great *Black* doctor of notoriety. The truth of the matter is that the first Doctor of *any* distinction was Imhotep from Africa (or **Alkebu-lan**) 5,000 years ago! He is regarded as the "father of medicine."

Our quest should be to return to our natural selves and become a self-thinking, self-sustaining and self-loving tribe once again. We must begin to function as God originally intended; as Black **Alkebu-lan** people, and dispense with the notion that we must be and act like others in order to be civilized, cultured, happy, wholesome, etc. . .{Incidentally, "Africa" was not the only name that the ancients gave to the continent. According to the great historian, Dr. Yosef A.A. ben-Jochannan, they respectfully called our motherland, "**Alkebu-lan.**"}

So it is the *collective* us that will benefit from a fresh new outlook on Blackness. With a proper understanding of who we are and why we are, we will be fortified with all the necessary ingredients to come together *collectively;* rise, join, embrace and love our African selves once again. 80% of our problems can be traced in some way to our *collective* inability to view ourselves in a positive light. We will never solidify a tie with each other until we are psychologically tied to our past. As the *collective* is reunited with history and reason, we will not hesitate to do business with one another. We will not hesitate to serve one another. We would not hesitate to trust one another. Our past is our bond. Our *collective* future depends upon our understanding and acknowledgment of our *entire* past.

Historical awareness will help to unite and solidify the *collective*. However, on an individual front, each of us must come to a basic understanding of how the human mind works, and how *thought* is the launching pad of our every action! We will make major leaps forward when the collective recognizes that the individual thought process is critically important and become aware of its vital significance to our *every* undertaking. I have channeled most of this book to that end. An individual must know the brain, as the *collective* must know its roots, for the mind *is* the individual's root, as history is the root of the collective. Just as the *collective* will fall pitifully short of sanity without a working understanding of history, the *individual* with historical intelligence will yet flounder in misery without an understanding of the mind and how he or she may be the catalyst for most of their personal strife. We will affect the necessary changes in this realm when we realize that **ultimate power lies within our minds.** A knowledgeable mind is a cultivated, pro-active mind... a mind that will reach the pinnacle of higher reasoning that I so designate an **UNSHACKLED-MIND!**

FAREWELL TO SLAVERY

MY PEOPLE WERE ENSLAVED.
AND NOW I STAND FREE,
A TESTAMENT TO THEIR COURAGE,
STRENGTH AND DETERMINATION.
THEY REMOVED MANACLES FROM
THEIR ARMS AND LEGS… AS I HAVE
REMOVED THE SHACKLES FROM MY MIND.

Almas J. Sami'

1

FAREWELL TO SLAVERY

To emancipate means to set free. Abraham Lincoln signed the Emancipation Proclamation over one-hundred fifty years ago. And with that signing, and later the passing of the 13th Amendment of the Constitution, came an end to slavery, at least on paper or by law. African Americans were free to do as they chose. The problem was that most Blacks never really saw themselves as freed men and women. They knew that White racists were still very much in control of Black folks lives and destinies.

However, the primary reason Africans were not truly free is that they still viewed themselves through the eyes of slaves. Their consciousness was still that of slaves. Were they all of a sudden proud of their Blackness just because they were "set free?" Of course not! They had been systematically taught for hundreds of years that Blackness was evil; Blackness was inferior; Blackness was second class.

They were even Bible-taught in such a manner that led them to believe that they were Black as a result of a curse from

God! Light skinned Blacks were psychologically separated from dark skinned Africans and made to feel "almost White," therefore, better than darker skinned brethren. Slaves were given a complete vocabulary of words that struck them down; nigger, coon, spear-chunker, etc. . . The list is virtually endless. So even though they were physically freed, their minds thus their actions remained that of slaves.

Bro. Haji Malik Shabazz, **(aka Minister Malcolm X)** outlined and explained this condition in a magnificent speech given at the London School of economics, (February 11, 1965): **"... we here in the West were made to hate Africa and hate the African. Why, the chain-reaction effect was it had to make us end up hating ourselves. You can't hate the roots of the tree without hating the tree, without ending up hating the tree ... We hated our African characteristics. We hated our African identity. We hated our African features. So much so that you would find those of us in the West who would hate the shape of our nose. We would hate the shape of our lips. We would hate the color of our skin and the texture of our hair."**

Bro. Shabazz spoke of the critical nature and importance of addressing and correcting these maladies over thirty years ago! Surely by now these topics should be the source of great debate among us Africans in America, yet we gloss over the problem and eventually go traipsing down that familiar road, the *"everything is the White mans' fault"* road. We must go back into our past and figure out what we did wrong — as well as reuse the things we did right! There were millions of Africans who refused to be slaves. They did not or could not "set" their minds to be slaves. Most of them died in rebellions. Others were killed while attempting to flee the wicked institution of subjugation. There were many slaves like **David Walker, Harriet Tubman, Frederick Douglass,** and the great Fula

Muslim Prince, **Abd Al-Rahman Ibrahima** who managed to use their minds to set their bodies free.

They were just like every other slave in body, however, their minds were as free as any man or woman who walked the streets of that era. That is what set the free African people apart from slaves; **STRONG, CULTIVATED MINDS!** They refused to see themselves and other Africans as niggers, coons and second class humans. Their minds were free long before they managed to set their bodies free. Sadly, slavery was so physically brutal and spiritually crippling that few Africans could make the journey to psychological freedom.

Look around today, you can still see remnants of the slave mentality! How often have you heard Blacks refer to themselves and other Blacks as "niggas?" Psychologists tell us that the words and language we use reflect what we truly feel on the inside. Never in the history of Africa did we refer to ourselves as niggas until our slave masters reprogrammed our minds to ready us to become slaves!

We were forced to internalize the notion that we were "sub-human niggas" during slavery. The sooner we began to accept as fact that we were niggas, the better suited for slavery we had become. It has been over one-hundred twenty years since we were "set free" yet we still refer to ourselves in the same manner that slave masters did yesterday… could it be that many of us still feel like second class humans today?

Will we need to get permission from "masa charlie" before we stop visualizing ourselves as niggas? When will we realize that slavery thoughts, or in other words, the mindsets of that era were simply bogus notions that were thrust upon us by unenlightened, slothful people who took us after we sold ourselves to them to perform labor that they were too lazy to do for themselves!

In order for the slavery system to be fully operational, we had to be sold on the notion or lie that we were niggas or innately beneath our slave masters. The sad fact that most Blacks still believe themselves to be niggas lends sad testimony to the harsh reality that we are still looking through lenses of slavery. Why do we still continue to view ourselves as second class citizens today? Perhaps it is because we have yet to undo those old backward thinking patterns:

NO NOT A NIGGA!

NO, NOT NIGGA, AFTER THESE MANY YEARS,
NO PERSON HAS YET RISEN TO DIVULGE YOU!
NO, NOT A NIGGA.

NO, NOT SECOND CLASS. NO, NOT DUMB.
NOT SLOW OF THOUGHT, NOT INBORN INFERIOR,
NOT LESS THAN WHOLE . . .
NO, NOT A NIGGA.

NOT OF LESS VALUE, NOT UNHOLY, NOT ON THE
DOWN SIDE, NOT UNDER, NOT ON THE BOTTOM,
NO, NOT A NIGGA.

SLAVE YOU ARE NO MORE, YET YOU HAVE NOT
BEEN TOLD, SO NIGGA YOU
THINK; KILL YOURSELF,
YOU WILL. HARM YOURSELF, YOU
WILL. CURSE YOURSELF,
YOU WILL, FOR YOU BELIEVE OF NIGGA.
YOU KNOW NOT MORE THAN THAT!

POVERTY CLAIMS YOU. CONFUSION
ENGULFS YOUR IDLE
INTELLECT. MISERY PERMEATES YOUR
UNCLAIMED SOUL. FOR YOU
BELIEVE NIGGA EXISTS
. . . YOU KNOW NOT OTHERWISE.

NO, YOU KNOW NOT YOURSELF.
YOU KNOW NOT YOUR

MOTHER, OR FATHER, OR YOUR
SONS AND DAUGHTERS.
FOR NIGGA THEY ARE NOT! EXCEPT
IN YOUR CHATTEL LACED
CONTEMPLATIONS . . .NO, NOT NIGGA!
NOT IN YOUR GODS' EYE . . . NO!

Almas J. Sami'

Life for us on this earth will never be complete until we collectively reach back and pick up the broken pieces of our past. We must once and for all come to know who we were before we were enslaved. Ask the average Black what we were before coming to this land, and you will find that we mistakenly believe we were little more than monkeys swinging from tree to tree!

Once I had a conversation with an elderly Black man about the inventions and contributions made by our people. After listening to my chatter for a while, he interrupted me and said, "Even so, the Blacks who invented these things had to get all their previous knowledge from Whites! The White man did everything!"

This Brother is trapped in a world that leads him to believe that everything evolves around, or came from White people! Naturally, with that faulty point of view, he felt himself and all Blacks to be naturally inferior to Whites. So, to him it was not necessarily a put down to be called a nigga! Deep down within every fiber of his being he believed he was a nigga!! The strangest and most wretched of humans are the ones who see themselves through the eyes of others... and who will deny the cold fact that we are a bizarre and pitiful lot? ***In our current state, we* are by choice!**

A closer look at our problems will reveal that inferior mindsets are shared by about eight out of ten African Americans in this country. That is why it hurts so much when we are disrespected by other races. We often "feel" humiliated as a result of our weakened mental state. It all comes down to the fact that we act and react according to what others believe or dictate. For instance, I was walking through a shopping center parking lot with a young brother man when a White woman quickly pressed her electric door locks as we walked by her car. This young brother was enraged and wanted to stop and let her have a piece of his mind. He wanted to let her know that she should not assume that all Black men were dangerous criminals. He was, to say the least beside himself with rage!

I found the whole incident humorous, which seemed to irritate him even more. He said, "Why are you laughing? Why do you take that bull#*$@! We don't have to let them put us down anymore." I told him that she didn't put me or him down. She couldn't have because she didn't know who we were. And even if she did know us, it is beyond my power and inclination to alter or change the way she felt about Blacks. It only matters what I think about me and other Blacks. We are all too sensitive about these matters. And as a consequence, we often end up chasing ghosts and other non-realities. We have the incredible ability to major in minor things!

I am much too busy with my day to day activities to stop and ponder over what some little White girl thinks about me or Blacks in general! I have places to go, people to see, and things to do. This brother allowed her to alter his whole evening! He wasn't able to enjoy himself for the rest of the day... all because a White thought of him as inferior, and it was too much to take. He allowed himself to be placed in a bad state of mind, and was really unable to do anything productive from that moment on!

Why are we "victimized" so easily? Well it goes right back to the sad fact that most of us *see* ourselves as niggas. We have distorted views and opinions of ourselves. Most of us really do not like the fact that we are members of the Black race! Let us just face this truth once and for all! Let us penetrate the fog and finally come to grips with what really ails us. This brother was so enraged because deep down inside, he agreed with the young White girl's assessment of our race! On the surface it is easy to deny these facts. Yet when we delve into our true psyches, the reality of self-hatred is all too gripping. After all, deep down inside, do you really believe anyone actually wants to be a nigga?

Underneath it all is the undeniable fact that we are without knowledge of self! In other words, we are **"rootless and ungrounded."**

Until and unless we get our history straight, we will continue to hate ourselves, and therefore continue to feel the hurt of being disrespected by other races. In this world, you get what you expect. You are what you think. You cannot possibly respect yourself or other Africans if you mistakenly believe we are niggas ... nay will you command respect from other races. We must come to know our past. There is no getting around this bit of truth.

If we were to see ourselves through the eyes of our grand ancestors, we will began to feel their presence and will thus be able to draw from their magnificent power! History will give us the strong, steady foundation needed to see our ways through our difficulties. And we will stop viewing ourselves through the eyes of other races. We will be able to get on with the business of being humans and start taking care of the important things in life, like learning mathematics, trigonometry and the higher sciences, etc ... Some of us have recently discovered great things about our heritage. For centuries, we were taught that Europeans were the only innovators, and achievers. We felt that we were just along for the ride ... and thankful that we were so fortunate to take advantage of the wonders that Whites brought about. (Masa sho is smart!)

We did not know that Africans were the first humans to walk on this earth! We were not taught that a place called Egypt was really named Kemet and was inhabited by Black African people ... our pyramid building, Black African ancestors! **(The name "Egypt" was given to Kemet by a conqueror from Greece whose name was "Aegyptos ... moreover,**

people from Kemet also called them- selves "Hamitu and were of the Anu Tribe.") Yes, civilization as we know it today was brought into existence by our ancient African fore parents.

We ushered in the sciences, mathematics, and the arts. Investigate the mind blowing book, **"The Ankh: African Origin of Electro-magnetism"** by **Nur Ankh Amen** and find out how our magnificent ascendants discovered and utilized electricity over 4,000 years ago!

If you find this fact hard to believe, then ponder the fact that we cannot today with all of our technology figure out how the pyramids were built, in fact, we do not have the brain power or know how to build a great pyramid today! Our people laid the foundations that have ushered us to modern day engineering and physics, thereby making space shuttles and other contemporary technologies a reality. We are so conditioned to think of ourselves as second class that these notions, indeed these truths, offend the senses!

There are hardly any innovations today that were not revelations of our ancestors of yesteryear! **All** roads lead through Kemet! By studying Kemet, we find a grand civilization that shines a magnificent light on the past, present and the future. We discover that she rose from Nubia into a grand civilization that baffles our weak and feeble minds of today. And in her fall, she cast a mighty eclipse over all of humankind as we know it. The fact of the matter is, had Kemet not fallen, humankind would be much farther advanced in the sciences than we are at the present!

For instance, Kemetian scientist were making grand strides in the study of aeronautics over two thousand years ago! **(A glider was found in Sakkora, Kemet in 1898, but since the European "discoverers" did not know what it was, it was dismantled and placed in the basement of a museum!)** Innovations such as these were thwarted as Kemet fell, and less knowledgeable people from Persia and Greece came into power. How much farther would we have been by now, had these great scientist from the motherland not been interrupted by the downfall of their world? Perhaps the Star Trek movies would be a reality for us today!

All of todays' societies, here in America and abroad are yet primitive, because humankind lost grand sources of knowledge when Alkebu-lan slowly declined and the great temples and universities, (such as at Waset, Kemet) which contained thousands of volumes of information collected over thousands and thousands of years were destroyed by savage brutes from other lands... ponder that truth, and you will get a new lease on life!

Furthermore, many contemporary inventions like the telephone transmitter, the stoplight, the gas mask, the shoemaking machine and many, many other innovations were born of African minds! Important medical discoveries and techniques, including open heart surgery were first successfully performed by persons of African descent. What a difference it makes when one is aware of one's own history. The mind shackles fall by the wayside!

A people will instinctively accomplish whatever they believe they have the inborn capacity to execute. For instance, if we knew that Africans conceived mathematics, we would more readily comprehend and rise to the challenges of math in school today. We would know that learning math is "natural." This is not to suggest that all Africans would excel in the higher sciences, but we would approach our studies with a different attitude... perhaps more zeal as our feelings of belonging elevates. This is why it is so vitally important for each and every Black person in this world to come to grips with their true and proper heritage.

I am often asked, "How did history get turned upside down?" I use the following illustration to clarify what happened: **Let us suppose there is a man who teaches himself to build a one story building. Later, he would teach his son the sum of all he has learned over the years. His son would then expand upon the knowledge left by the father and naturally teach himself even more until he has learned to construct a two story structure. As time passes, he would funnel all of his accumulated knowledge to his daughter. She would grasp his know-how and cultivate even more knowledge until she has mastered the construction of a three story edifice. This natural progression would continue for many generations until the family has learned to erect majestic pyramids!**

Now let us suppose that another family comes into the picture. They are taught the accumulated lessons and become somewhat proficient at constructing buildings. A few generations later, the second family kills the remaining knowledgeable members of the first family and removes the blueprints and all the acquired knowledge to another location far away. The only surviving members of the first family were ones who were not yet taught how to con- struct. The first family is now left without essential knowledge, while the second family continues the growth procession based upon the accumulated knowledge acquired from the ancient members of family number one.

The first family is now without a foundation or roots! As the years go by, certain members of family number two reconstructs history and convinces the first family that they have always been without know-how and will continue to decline because they are genetically inferior. They learn that they do not have the inborn capacity to construct buildings. You can imagine what happens after many generations of ignorance and misinformation. The first family will at some point begin to behave in a peculiar

way as they are cut off from the truth about themselves. Their minds become shackled and they will begin to worship family number two! They would hate themselves and love family number two. They would actually strive to be more like family number two!

This is exactly what happened to our people. We are the original thinkers of the world, yet in our pitiful state we linger behind others who have built themselves up with our ancestors' expertise and experience. **{When you see museums displaying so-called "Egyptian artifacts", you are in fact viewing a part of your own heritage and culture.** *These museum items were "stolen" from our fallen peoples!* **If anyone tells you otherwise, they are simply lying and hiding the truth. Actually, if you stepped back from the situation for a moment and thought it through logically, you would quickly come to the conclusion that it is absurd to believe that dark skinned, nappy headed, big-lipped White people ruled Kemet, Alkebu-lan over five thousand years ago!}**

In our shackled state, we will honor the names of family number two. We will straighten our hair, lighten our skin and curse our God-given traits. If the truth would be known, in our heart of hearts, we strive to become members of family number two! This process began long before we were stolen from the motherland. It is all based upon the fact that we are without knowledge of ourselves... our past is not a part of us! African tribalism, which insured our separation, coupled with European misinformation were the distinct ingredients needed to shackle our minds for generations.

This is precisely the vice that goes to the core of our problems. We are unthinking people, because slave masters rendered us incapable of self-generated thought. This process was known as **"seasoning".** Slaves had to endure an orientation process to ready themselves for the special brand of hell they were thrown into! They had to be seasoned to think negative, crippling thoughts so that their resistance to the system would be minimized.

Unfortunately, we are today still grappling with those mindsets that were carved into our recent ancestors' minds. We are still seasoned to believe we are niggas. We are seasoned to believe that we must conk our hair. We are still seasoned to think that black skin is ugly. We are still seasoned to believe it is not weird to wear the names of other races. We will remain seasoned until we decide to make the psychological changes to rid ourselves of past thinking patterns. The first step in curing an ailing patient is to get that patient to recognize as fact that they are ill. The second step is to get them to believe they have the power and wherewithal to properly deal with their maladies or illness. My people, we are desperately, near terminally ill; Black man, Black woman; heal thyself!

How many times have you heard light skinned Blacks belittling dark skinned Blacks for being "too Black?" And what do we mean when we talk about "good hair" and "bad hair?" These are graphic examples of how far African Americans need to go to attain psychological freedom! **WHEN WILL WE LET GO OF SLAVERY?** Ole' Abe Lincoln reluctantly removed the shackles from our bodies, however, we must come to the realization that our minds can only be unshackled by *us*! When will *we* unshackle *our* minds? When will *we* realize that *we* are family number *one*?

(By referring to us as family number one, I am in no way suggesting that we are superior. I am merely stating that we are older and have a lot of tradition to bring to the table... traditions and birthrights that lay far outside the realm of our experiences and accomplishments in this land called the United States of America!)

Somehow, I feel our enslaved ancestors who were brought to America are disappointed at so many of us who choose not to think for ourselves. They did not always have such choices. Their minds were shackled because their hands and legs were shackled. Today our hands and legs are shackled because our minds are shackled!

We curse White racists on the one hand, while continuing to use their words and rhetoric to define ourselves on the other hand! Freedom comes from within. African Americans collectively have yet to make that journey to free ourselves mentally. We need to understand that slave thoughts hold us back much more than White racists ever could. **We must stop using their mindsets and words of hatred to define ourselves.**

I will never forget the look on the face of one of my friends from Alkebu-lan when he asked me why a Black American called him a nigga while they were socializing together. How could I explain to him that we regularly use that word to define ourselves... we have done so since slavery? This slave mentality affects us at every turn. As a result of these slave mindsets, some Africans in this country look down their noses at Africans from Africa. Why is this true? Well, it has been that way since before the end of slavery. American born slaves considered themselves to be superior to newly arriving Africans. This was as a result of the mind shackling process. Everything Black or African was to be shunned. Slaves were rewarded for being anti-Black and anti-African. Lies became truths... and truths became lies. What we thought was up was really down. We would face west looking for a sunrise! Will we stop thinking negatively of ourselves? I remember how Black pride swelled in the sixties when James Brown sang the words, "I'm Black and I'm Proud." We all got caught up in those words. Many of us accepted Blackness as beautiful. We would do well to capture those same feelings with the intent to unshackle our minds.

It would not be difficult! We should use the positive examples of powerful Black leaders, entertainers and activists. What would happen if African Americans viewed themselves as equals? What would be the result of masses of Africans deciding once and for all to defiantly escape from our slave thought patterns? We would elevate our esteem as individuals and as a people.

I am happy to report that it is happening all over the country. If you would stop and listen, you could hear mind shackles hitting the ground. We are emerging! We are at the daybreak of understanding! There are African American lecturers, authors and activists cropping up all over the place. There is a network of Black-owned bookstores supporting them. We are beginning to come together and exchange positive information about our heritage. Young brothers and sisters have turned the music industry into a channel through which they can educate or "rap" to other youth. I have heard some powerful messages presented through some "rap" music. Our airwaves are filled with the all important messages of self-love and self-determination. The greats: Oscar Michaeux, Melvin Van Peebles, Spike Lee, Ava DuVernay, Tyler Perry, Antoine Fuqua, and Ryan Kyle Coogler to name a few has given birth to a host of young directors and producers of cinema who are literally changing the way Black youths view themselves! There are countless other great minds! Who is better to pull the wagon of knowledge to us than Ivan Van Sertima, Maulana Karenga, Charles Finch, or Asa G. Hilliard?

You may think there is not much you could do as an individual to make a difference. However, nothing could be farther from the truth. Refuse to take part in those slavery pity parties where we get together and exchange stories of how the "White man" is holding us back. Get rid of that slave thought. If not, you will be forever held in bondage in the recesses of your own mind. I am not suggesting that racism is nonexistent; however, there is plenty of self- cleansing and self-reevaluation that we must take care of first. We spend far too much time worrying about the "White man." **We should make ourselves a priority, for a change!**

WE MUST COME TO THE REALIZATION THAT THERE IS NOTHING INHERENTLY WRONG WITH US. WE MUST FINALLY LEARN THAT THERE IS NOTHING WRONG WITH OUR LIPS. WE MUST LEARN THAT THERE IS NOTHING WRONG WITH OUR KINKY HAIR. WE MUST LEARN THAT THERE IS NOTHING WRONG WITH OUR SKIN TONES, IN ALL OF OUR MAJESTIC SHADES! Know that God did not create "niggas," Slave masters made "niggas." It is a big lie... do not subscribe to it. You are a child of God on equal terms and footing with the rest of God's children.

Study our history — I recommend that you start with the work of **Maulana Karenga,** Introduction to Black Studies; **Na'im Akbar,** Chains And Images of Psychological Slavery; **Molefi Asante,** Kemet, Afrocentricity, and Knowledge. And for youth studies, **Jawanza Kunjufu,** Lessons From History A Celebration in Blackness; **Baba Zak Kondo,** A Crash Course In Black History: 150 Important Facts About Afrikan Peoples.

There are many other great individuals who have chronicled the history of Africans and African Americans). The late **Drusilla Dunjee Houston's** powerful book, "Wonderful Ethiopians of the Ancient *Cushite Empire*" will leave you bursting with pride! And if your desire is to completely purge your mind of historical inaccuracies, you must unquestionably, absolutely "study" the works of the late great West African scientist, **Cheikh Anta Diop**! Specifically his masterpiece titled, *"Civilization or Barbarism."* And for added stimulation, rap your mind around the powerful work of **Charles Finch's** *The African Background to Medical*

Science. Or perhaps **Yosef A.A. Ben-Jochannan's,** "Black Man of the Nile." You will discover how your Alkebu-lan kinfolk's planted the seeds of civilization.

You have a rich, proud heritage. Stand tall and face the world on equal footing. Bow down to no one. Find out who you are, then set out to stake your claim in the world. The world is yours to do with as you think. Just grab your mind, mold your mind, change your outlook where it needs to be changed. Educate yourself! Ex- amine your thoughts! Ask yourself some critical questions. What are your concepts about life? Why do you have those concepts? The answers to life lies in your thinking! Free yourself! Unshackle your mind! The free-world awaits you!

ROAR WITH THE LIONS

I HEAR THE ROARS OF THE GREAT ONES.
THEIR MIGHTY DECLARATIONS REACH UP
FROM THE PAST AND PRESENT;

BESTOWING POWERFUL NUGGETS
OF WISDOM AND KNOWLEDGE.

MY PLACE IS WITH THE LIONS!

Almas J. Sami'

2

ROAR WITH THE LIONS

Contrary to common belief, most great men and women endured many heartbreaks and were forced to overcome great obstacles while on their upward climb. It is not accurate to suggest, however, that setbacks are desirable! The difference between those who roar and those who whimper lie in their mental approaches to life's ups and downs. Great thinking people have acquired the ability to simply view life's ups and downs in a different light. They control their thinking rather than allow their circumstances to determine their mental outlook.

In order to become "great", a person must learn to utilize the gift of "thought" to change the face of things. Hard luck offers us the opportunity to grow and develop, **(provided we learn from our mistakes).** Great thinking people realize this vital truth long before they are recognized as being great. Take time to study the lives and philosophies of great thinkers. Put your own problems aside long enough to acquaint yourself with the lives of great leaders, inventors, educators and achievers. Pay particular attention to their early years before they reached acclaim. You will find that they had experienced what you may be experiencing now... grief, confusion and pain, and yet have a burning desire to make a change; to grow, to become more.

Booker T. Washington and Frederick Douglass were born into slavery. Martin Luther King, Jr. had his doubts early on. Marva Collins struggled to get her school going. James Earl Jones stuttered. Maya Angelou tasted defeat many times. Yet they all endured, learned and became great! They fulfilled their dreams! You may think you are down and out, but through your study of great people you will discover that you are not alone. You do not hold a monopoly on pain, failure and anguish. With the right thought control applied, you will see better days!

Frederick Douglass was not "born" great. He sacrificed and made himself great. When he was a child, he had a burning desire to learn to read and write. But there was this one problem; it was against the law to teach a slave to do such. Douglass did not let that deter him. He was clever enough to trick White kids into teaching him. He would point out a letter or word to them that he did not know. However, instead of asking them what the word was, he would merely mispronounce it. For instance, if he saw the word "shoe", he would ask, "Is that word 'see'?" The White kids would laugh and say "no dummy, that word is shoe!" You see, Douglass knew that was the only way in which he could enlist their assistance. He learned a great deal by letting them ridicule him in this manner. He ignored their insults, and just kept asking "dumb" questions! Brother Douglass went on to surpass them to become one of the great orators and literary minds of his day!

I need only mention Ray Charles and Stevie Wonder to make a resounding point: Your setbacks and obstacles are really and truly your opportunities for greatness! You must learn to look beyond that which appears to be reality, and find the true causes that affect your life. Usually, the answers to our questions lie beneath the surface. Life has presented you with the opportunity to crystallize your thoughts toward greatness! Now you have the chance to take setbacks and make comebacks! You can turn it all around through the process of thought control.

You can be assured of the fact that all of the other great people like yourself "took their shots." The mighty lions went through growth periods when their loud roars were nothing more than weak, seemingly insignificant purrs. Yet they endured these times until they learned to utilize the inborn power of the mind. When you stop and think about it, you will realize that is what America is all about — the freedom to choose and direct one's thinking! But you, and you alone must choose how you use the power of thought.

Sure you have been discriminated against; probably too many times to mention. But how many times have you slammed the golden door of opportunity in your own face because you simply "thought" these negative conditions existed! If you would stop and analyze the facts, you may learn that the situation may have been worsened by your mental outlook or faulty psychological conditioning.

You have the freedom of thought. Thought is the essence of what we bring into this world. Indeed, thought is life! When you are fully aware of this golden secret, you will cherish your every thought. You will also carefully choose your thoughts. You will realize that it is your God-given **responsibility** to think properly and constructively. No matter how bad you view your situation, there is sure to be someone out there who is overcoming more challenging obstacles than you are currently facing. Every time you get the urge to host a pity party for yourself, just stop for a moment and reflect upon the atrocities that your ancestors endured in this country during slavery. What would they think about your crying over our petty concerns of today? **John W. Blassingame** chronicled slave life in his powerful book entitled, **"The Slave Community,"** in which he gave chilling illustrations of the things that our people had to tolerate. You will learn that many of our people died for the rights and freedoms that we take for granted today?

Do not allow ups and downs, discrimination, hatred or anything else to rob you of your right to choose your thoughts. Great people already know this truth, that is why they are great. They first became great thinkers! Know that all circumstances are actually presented to you for your own benefit. Even if it does not "appear" to be so at first glance. You must make personal growth a priority in your life. Everything that has happened to you thus far is of some benefit. You cannot reap the benefits of growth through circumstance until you decide to view your present state or condition in a positive light. The phrase, "growth through circumstance" simply means that you acquire the insight to look for the positive in every situation. No matter what happens, you will have the ability to make mental adjustments, so that you can learn from the event — or even turn the negative situation into a positive one.

Count your blessings! Literally list on a sheet of paper the blessings you now have. Can you walk? Can you talk? Can you think? List them all! Then stop taking your present assets for granted. Focus on, and start appreciating your blessings. Why, the fact that you can read the words on this page is of a great advantage to you. Great lions that came before you paid the ultimate sacrifice for your privilege to read and write! Stop! Think! And rejoice at the thought of your present day advantages. If you listen carefully, you will be able to hear your ancestors celebrating the very fact that you are here, and you have a chance to go places, to do things and become what they dreamed you would someday become.

Take inventory of what you have now and start from there. You cannot began to make gains until you are in a good frame of mind. But, you cannot get in a good frame of mind *consistently*, until you learn to appreciate whatever assets you have at the present! You must strive for consistency, so that you will be better able to alleviate mood swings and bouts of depression. You will discover that things are not as bad as you first "thought" they were. You must have an appreciation of where you are now before you can even begin to formulate a vision for a better day.

Look around you! There are sure to be a host of blessings already bestowed upon you. Look at this country. Your ancestors help build this great land. Millions of Africans and African Americans gave the ultimate sacrifice for the rights and freedoms you can now enjoy. Accept that fact! Think positively about your health, or the health of your family. Look for and find thoughts that are positive. Why is this important? Well, if your ultimate goal is to grow and achieve, does it not make since that you could grow easier and faster if you are in a firm, positive state of mind? Of course it does! If you are presently encountering hardship, by all means, stop and allow yourself a period of grief. But resolve to move on!

Remember that there are few hardships today that would even remotely compare to the ones suffered by our ancestors. So for their sake, get your act together! Resolve to build upon the foundations they laid by the sweat of their brow! Intentionally become a happy person. If you are happy most of the time, you will begin a chain reaction. Other positive circumstances will make them- selves available to you! It is nature's law! As Bobby McFerrin says, "Don't Worry, Be Happy." The fact of the matter is, your negative or unwanted conditions are present in part because of your ignorance of nature's "thought laws."

There is no situation that cannot be of value to you now or maybe at a future date. Great people are aware of this age old truth. But they did not learn these truths until they experienced and felt what you may be feeling and experiencing now. Like you, they had a strong desire to overcome their conditions or circumstances — and themselves!

So cherish your every moment regardless of who and what you are. Remember, as you began to count your blessings, you will feel better. When you feel better, you will think better thoughts. When you think better thoughts, you will automatically attract more desirable conditions! Last but certainly not least, you will act better. It is very important to remember to be patient. Give nature a chance to operate. Meanwhile, enjoy the scenery! Take your rightful place among the great lions! When your time comes, you will let out a mighty roar!

PERCEPTIONS

I MAKE MY WORLD!
I CANNOT ALWAYS CHOOSE
THE CIRCUMSTANCES, YET I DO
CONTROL HOW THOSE
CIRCUMSTANCES AFFECT ME.
TO BE AND FUNCTION
AS I THINK PROPER, FREE FROM THE BONDAGE
OF VIEWING MY LIFE
THROUGH THE EYES OF OTHERS . . .
IT'S MY GOD-GIVEN PRIVILEGE
TO SEE WHAT I SEE.
I SEE A CHOICE… MY CHOICE!
I CHOOSE TO NAVIGATE MY THOUGHTS!

Almas J. Sami'

3

PERCEPTIONS

How do you frame your world? How do you "view" yourself within that frame? Perhaps other people would view your world or your circumstances in a different vein than you do. It all depends on how you "perceive" or "see" things.

Many times your perceptions will determine your opinions or actions. Suppose you were walking down the street and saw a sixty year old man with his arms around a thirty year old woman. What would you think? Is he an older man with a young wife or girl- friend? Or could he simply be a loving father showing affection towards his daughter? What you perceive the situation to be will determine your thoughts, or it will color your "view." Perhaps it would be wise to examine some of your present perceptions.

Is this exercise a simple little "mind game" or could it perhaps shed light on how you view your world? Maybe you have preconceived ideas about how African people are to be or perform. Many of us are handicapped because of what we perceive Blackness to be! For example, suppose I were to ask you to describe a businessman between ages sixty and seventy. What picture do you see in your mind? What if I said the man was very rich; one of the most successful businessmen in the country. Would you envision a man that looked like George Bush, or did you see one resembling John Johnson, publisher of Ebony Magazine... one of the wealthiest men in the country? How and what you perceive Black people to be will greatly affect your attitude about Blackness. More important, it reflects how you "see" yourself in your world.

Reexamine the way you view your world and open your mind to the endless array of positive people and circumstances that exists in the world. You may have overlooked great opportunities in the past if your perception has been faulty. Perhaps losing that job was a blessing in disguise. Maybe if you looked around you would discover a great opportunity lying in the wake. Maybe there is a service that is needed that you could provide. If you would but commit yourself to servicing your fellow brothers and sisters in some valuable capacity, you would completely wipe out any mental damage done as a result of having to put up with the discrimination that we are forced to face while working for others.

SEEK TO GO INTO BUSINESS FOR THYSELF! OFFER GOOD SERVICE TO OTHERS AND YOU WILL BE BOM- BARDED WITH THE OPPORTUNITY TO BECOME SELF- SUSTAINING!

I have a friend who had his car repaired by a mechanic from Viet- nam who came to this country a few years ago. Not only did he do a fantastic job of repairing the auto, but he was so inclined to serve that he followed up his work with a phone call a week later to make sure that his work was satisfactory... despite the fact that he lived over 90 miles away from my friend! Our Vietnam friend is committed to service. His business is overflowed with referrals from satisfied customers! It is a sure bet that there are opportunities waiting for you to pluck them as you would fresh fruit from the vineyard, but you must first pluck negative and crippling thoughts from your mind!

However, opportunities are often hidden. They are only visible to clear thinking, mentally-focused people. Rather than mope resentfully or sulk over a lost job, you could focus on new possibilities. They are always present, but you cannot see them if you are in a bad frame of mind. Your frame of mind can affect or color your perceptions, thus making it difficult to "see" or take advantage of opportunities that may be right under your nose! You are what you see, and you see what you think! So what if you were fired because you are Black. Decide to control your thinking. If we perceive our lives to be harder because we are Black, then those are the signals that we will send to our brain. It affects the way we think, therefore, the way we feel and act. It would be more psychologically advantageous for you to consider your life to be more "challenging" rather than "harder."

Our behavior is affected either positively or negatively depending on how we think and feel.There are foreigners who come to America and do very well in business. It is because they perceive America to be the land of opportunity. No one told them that the odds were "stacked" against them.

We can change the way we represent life to ourselves, and instantly, we can see life differently. We see opportunities right in front of us that were there all along. We can "color" life anyway we want. I have often heard Blacks say that we have to be twice as good as White people in order to survive on the job or in sports. Well, that may or may not be true, but the question is, what is wrong with disciplining yourself to be "twice as good?" Super successful people in every walk of life will tell you they had to be better than the next guy. That was their outlook; a driving principle that elevated them to great heights!

Susan Taylor of Essence Magazine had her work cut out when she decided to venture into the publishing business. Publishing a magazine expressly for Black women was considered a risky venture. But this brilliant sister decided to make herself twice as good! No one today could deny that she is a resounding success. So what you may perceive to be a handicap is actually a principle of success! If you decide to commit yourself to that principle; to be twice as good as everyone else, you would soar on to greatness in your chosen field. It all depends on how you "view" life!

The world is full of achievers who decided to make themselves "twice as good." Michael Jordan is arguably "twice as good" as other basketball players — at least he strives to be. The great general Colon Powell sat out as a young Army Lieutenant to make himself better than everyone else. There is not doubt that he accomplished this task and reached his goals. His autobiography, "My American Journey" is a great read from a great man. The gigantic writer, Toni Morrison, has unquestionably set standards that few if any could ever reach. She is monumental because her mindset is monumental!

What are your perceptions? Can you do anything? Are there limits placed on your expectations based on faulty perceptions? Open your mind to endless possibilities! Challenge your representations of your world! How do we form faulty perceptions? Well, the most direct way is through our past experiences. Often, we get caught up in the past and do not allow ourselves to get free of those negative encounters. Many times we experience racial discrimination at our work environments or schools. After continually running into that foolishness we give up. We lose hope. If those negative experiences go unchecked, they, like every other negative emotion, tend to grow and fester like a cancer.

Soon, negativism touches and stains every endeavor that you pursue, every venture that you undertake… until you reach a stage where your inner and outer world is so tainted that you will swear up and down that the world is against you and the "White man" is spending every waking hour of his life trying to devise new ways to hold you down. However, if you were of the proper thought-set, your mind would constantly be on the look out for opportunity. You would eagerly confront and conquer most of the silly racism that we encounter.

Warren Moon, a hall of fame quarterback, is a classic example of what happens when one uses gut determination and vision to overcome racial obstacles. Most people do not know that Moon was rejected time after time while on his upward march to becoming one of the premier quarterbacks in the National Football League. He was a standout player in high school. Yet he was told that he did not have the talent to make it in major college football. He had to go to a junior college in order to "prove" himself.

Later, the University of Washington gave him a scholarship. He went on to set school records and was voted the Most Valuable Player of his conference. His troubles did not end there, however, for he was told by the professional scouts that he did not possess the skills to play the quarterback position in the National Football League! They said that his arm was not strong enough. The aver- age person would have quit right there... but not Moon! He kept his head up, and went to play for the Canadian Football League. After "improving" himself and becoming the most prolific Quarterback in CFL history, he was highly recruited by several NFL teams. He signed with the Houston Oilers for the highest salary ever paid to a professional football player at the time! His determination paid off!

Whenever we experience these racial situations, we must deal with them immediately. How do we deal with it? Well, it is not always easy but it is always very simple.

First we need to understand what happens psychologically. Usually when we encounter discrimination, we tend to take it personally. And by doing so, we give undo importance to this ungodly happening. We have been conditioned since slavery to react to White racist assaults, (both physical and verbal assaults). I am not a believer in "*cheek-turning*" ... one must meet physical force with a greater force! However, we must refrain from getting blown off course because of White racist rhetoric or words. Their words of hatred are mere words, and are in no way worth paying the least bit of attention to ... so get on with your life!

We have to remember that prejudiced people are really very small, simple-minded people. They suffer from an acute inferiority complex. They feel badly about themselves. There is a saying, "your view of the world is a reflection of yourself." In other words, a person can only give what they have and feel inside. If they have hatred for themselves, they have only hatred to give to the world. The same is true vice versa. If they have true love for themselves, they give only true love to their fellow men and women. What does "*true*" love mean? True self-love recognizes the purpose for love ... to give freely to the world. The natural laws of love are first and foremost of all other laws of nature. In order to understand self-love, one must have an understanding of true love — **LOVE IS GOD!**

Just think how backwards a person has to be in order to hate an entire race of Gods' creation. They are out of touch with who they are ... a simple child of God whose function is to serve God and creation. Imagine the hatred one must feel toward himself if he is at odds with himself, his world and his God. His mind and heart are not aligned with nature.

I have never met a racist (Black or White) who is happy with himself or the world. These people are to be pitied. Feel sorry for them, because they are surely hurting. Take no pleasure in another person's pain and anguish. But by the same token, do not let a pitiful racist color your world with the same misery that they are feeling. Refuse to give them the power to affect the way you feel about yourself or your world. Get rid of the negative baggage, or otherwise it will change or affect the way you view yourself and your circumstances in life. It can take away your ability to focus on your goals at hand.

Not all White people are racist. Study the lives of great Black people. Many of them will tell you of White friends who helped them along. El-Hajj Malik El-Shabazz, aka Minister Malcolm X was aided by "White" Muslims while on his historic pilgrimage to Mecca. Were it not for the assistance from some of his White Muslim friends, he may not have been able to make that life-changing journey. Look at what Cus D'Amato did for Mike Tyson. Iron Mike will tell you that Cus was a remarkable man. Tyson's short-lived downfall was aided and abetted by both Black leeches as well as White sharks! It is just as ridiculous to assume that all Whites will hinder your progress as it is to presume that all Blacks will automatically assist you. Let go of the faulty perception that all White people are racist. It is simply not true. How many times have you *perceived* ghosts of discrimination where there in fact were none?

Refuse steadfastly to let a racist hold you back from being all that you can be. You must start with the racist that dwells within your own mind and heart. Secondly, it is critical that you keep and harbor a healthy perception of yourself. That being the case, your whole world will change! Your outlook of yourself should be a positive one. Perceive yourself to be a cherished child of God. The better you feel about yourself, the better you will feel about your world. The process of reshaping perceptions requires that you re-shape situations to enable you to look at a potential baleful circumstance in a more positive light.

For instance, suppose you were turned down for a job for reasons you "perceive" to be discriminatory. The first thing to do is realize there is nothing wrong with you or your color. *(If you know your Black history, this step is easy.)* Secondly, remember that racists are really sad pathetic people who feel hatred for themselves. Now here is the clincher: **Forgive that sad, pathetic person. Do Not Hold A Grudge; If you focus on your negative feelings about the racist, you will drain yourself of valuable energy... hate or resentment takes away your ability to think clearly. Therefore, you must forgive racist people... for your own sake as well as theirs!**

If you maintain a fresh open attitude, and keep trying, the right job in the right place at the right time will become available. Be "thankful" that you did not get the job, because you did not want to work with a racist anyway! Then immediately continue the search for the right job or may be a perfect business opportunity. It is quite simple — not necessarily easy, but it is very simple! Laws of nature dictate that right thinking people will get exactly what they need. It is nature's law! Perceptions are simply the way you choose to color your world. However, you can only have the proper outlook by choice. The ball is always in your court!

YOUR MIND, YOUR GUIDANCE SYSTEM

MY MIND IS THE SHAPER OF MY WORLD, AS I AM THE SHAPER OF MY MIND.

Almas J. Sami'

4

YOUR MIND, YOUR GUIDANCE SYSTEM

Our minds are the most powerful instruments in this universe. With our minds we can (and do) shape our futures. Set your mind on a direction, and it will pull you towards an end result.

For instance, if you have ever smoked cigarettes, you will agree with me when I say that cigarettes are nasty tasting, nasty smell- ing and truly disgusting! Even if you presently smoke, you will agree with my assessment. Think back to the very first time you smoked a cigarette. Remember how it made you gag? Your nose burned, your eyes burned and you felt dizzy!

So why did you ever smoke another one? Were you trying to punish yourself? Did you enjoy that dizzy, sick feeling and just could not wait to experience it again? Of course not. You had already "set" your mind in motion. You had already given your mind the instructions to smoke cigarettes. Who knows why you decided to suck that stuff into your lungs. It could have been for a variety of reasons. Cigarette advertisements glamorized smoking. Advertisers know exactly how to capture the imagination with titillating images that made smoking seem "cool." Or maybe you knew some- one who smoked and you followed in their footsteps. Years ago, many so-called experts in the medical establishment actually pre- scribed cigarettes to "calm nerves!"

For whatever the reason, you decided to join the ranks of the smokers. Once your mind was "set" to smoke, you overcame the dizziness. You overlooked your burning nose. "So what's a little cough?" You fulfilled your desire. What is more, your mind was so strong that you soon found smoking pleasurable! Your mind accomplished what you wanted it to ... you became a smoker!

THE MIND DOES NOT REASON OR JUDGE, IT JUST DELIVERS! ONCE YOU UNDERSTAND THIS TRUTH, THE QUICKER YOU WILL GET A HANDLE ON THIS LIFE. IT IS YOUR MIND, LYING DORMANT, WAITING FOR EI- THER YOU OR SOMEONE ELSE TO SET IT ON THE DIRECTIONS THAT YOU WILL EVENTUALLY TAKE! If you decided to quit smoking, and your desire was strong enough, you "set" your mind to it and you eventually became a non-smoker. You decided it was a nasty, disgusting, filthy ordeal and you "set" your mind to get rid of the habit. You may have joined a quit smoking club, or organization. You may have gradually cutback, or if your "mindset" was strong enough, you just quit "cold turkey." If you set your mind to become more physically fit, you did not gain a pound during the process of withdrawal from the nicotine.

The trick is to find a reason to quit that is stronger than your reason for smoking! I know of a man who quit when his wife said that kissing him was the equivalent of licking a wet ash tray! He quit that very moment! His embarrassment was stronger than his need for nicotine satisfaction. Even though nicotine is a dangerous narcotic, and extremely addictive, this brother was able to push the chemical dependency aside in a twinkling of an eye. There was no outside stimulus ... the only change that took place was the change of his mind! He found (however accidentally) something that was stronger than his chemical dependency. Once his mind discovered a new avenue, his life changed direction forever! It is amazing! The mind will pull you to wherever you truly "feel" you should be. What triggers "feeling?" Thoughts trigger feelings!

Our thoughts are like seeds. Plant thoughts of happiness and success ... success and happiness will be reaped. It is a law of nature. We all understand certain laws of nature. We know that if we jump from a tree the law of gravity will dictate that we will come down rather than go up. If we run head first into a brick wall, certain laws of pain will immediately come into effect! We should also learn that there are thought laws. Thought laws, like all natural laws, adhere to the rule of "cause and effect." This rule dictates that everything happens for a reason. Your thinking patterns are the precursors of the circumstances and situations in your life. **THOUGHTS GIVE BIRTH TO "THINGS!"**

For instance, if you were overweight (the effect) it would undoubtedly be because you ate too much of the wrong foods (the cause). It is simple. Why would a person's mindset be to get fat? It probably never was. Perhaps the mind is "set" to eat when that person "feels" depressed or anxious. Maybe their mind is "set" on bad eating habits. Often, eating gets linked up in our minds with other activities like reading or watching television. Whatever the case, the result is the same — overweight. You can see how cause and effect laws are ever-present. Everything happens for a reason.

Let us take the case of a little brother whom we will call Kunta. As Kunta is just a child, his mind is wide open to be "set" by his parents or his environment. These two factors will most likely give his life direction. Incredibly, psychologists tell us that we form 80% of our personality by the age of eight! By the time we are 18, we have already molded 95% of our values and outlooks in life! These are mind boggling statistics, especially when you consider that many parents believe children to be less important that adults. What if Kunta heard his mama constantly complain that Blacks just cannot make it in this country — that the White man will not let Blacks advance. "Life sho is hard on a nigga."

If Kunta hears this negative "life is unfair" talk long enough, he will begin to believe it. And by the time Kunta is a grown man, his mind is set on the idea (or lie) that he cannot succeed. So why should he attempt to set and attain worthy goals? He mistakenly "thinks" that White people are in control of his life; therefore, they are responsible for his life of repeated failures. It is a safe bet that his mama or daddy had the same experiences when they were children. That is exactly how and why we can have generations of African families fail, year after year, generation after generation. What would happen to Kunta if a more enlightened parent, a preacher, a banker or a respectable person implanted or "set" Kunta's mind towards success and happiness during those first critical eight years of his life? His chances of success and happiness would greatly increase. Even if Kunta's parents lived in a poor neighborhood, he would still most likely rise to success with the right "mindset."

Let us take the fantastic story of the internationally renowned Pediatric Neurosurgeon from John Hopkins Hospital, Doctor Ben Carson. This brother was not raised in a fabulous neighborhood with all of the comforts of life. Yet he was fortunate enough to have a stern, loving mother who constantly instilled pride and discipline in his young and impressionable mind. She believed in him and made sure that he believed in himself. Despite his early surroundings, he went on to become the first doctor to surgically separate Siamese twins! Even though his family was impoverished when he was a youth, his mother never let him use their financial situation as an excuse to be anything less than excellent. Even though they did not have money, they still had goals and dreams!

There is a huge difference between being "broke" and being "poor." A poor person is down and without hope — lost, discouraged and beaten. A broke person does not feel helpless or hopeless. They may be "broke" financially, but not mentally or spiritually "bro- ken." They still have a zest for life. They have goals. More important is the fact that they believe they have the ability to achieve their goals. They believe their present financial ailment is a temporary condition.

These are totally different mindsets. Your state of mind will deter- mine your state of affairs. If you are broke and unhappy, just reset your mind to be happy and successful. You can more easily do so by finding a way to serve your fellow brother man. Look for a goal that you would like to obtain and soon your whole life will change. He who controls his mind, controls his conditions and his world.

Look at Oprah Winfrey. She was a troubled youth whose mind was set toward success by her father. How many other Oprahs are out there... kids just ready to be launched in a positive direction? Oprah is a fine example for all of humankind! However, Oprah did have to buckle down and make a grand commitment. You can be assured that Oprah put in long hours. She undoubtedly had her share of setbacks, but she hung in there. She persevered. She was able to withstand heartbreak and setback because she had a positive mindset, backed by her belief system. I am sure there were many people that came to her aid along the way (both Black and White).

That is another one of natures' laws. If your conviction and dedication are strong enough, you almost magically attract the people and other resources to your aid! It is a snowball effect! I am sure Oprah encountered racism, but she is a living testimony to the fact that nothing can stand in the way of a mind that has been "set" to a given positive direction. The law works both positively and negatively. A person whose mind is set to smoke will overcome sickness and dizziness to fulfill that mindset. Likewise, you can overcome racism or any other element or condition and fulfill your minds desire.

The trick is to first find a worthy goal or ambition. If your want or desire is strong enough, your mind will takeover and "pull" you toward the thing you want. However, it is critically important that you examine your thoughts and mindsets. Challenge your every thought. If your thoughts are unworthy of your ambitions, get rid of those thoughts. If you are hanging around a non-supportive crowd, get a new crowd!

Study the life of some successful person that is living and doing what you want to do. Copy them exactly. Pretend you are doing those things. Feel the way you think you would feel if you were living your ideal life! Humans have remarkable abilities. If we act the way we would like to feel, we then feel the way we are acting! Your feelings always reflect what you think, and incredibly, you can alter the way you think by acting like whatever you imagine as appropriate. In other words, if you act successful, your thinking is thereby altered and you will eventually be successful as a result of the forward motion. What would you be like? How would you act?

Give your mind an exact picture to go by. For instance, suppose your goal is to become an attorney. You should find an attorney and discover what kind of person they are. What do they think? What did they study? How did they study? Where did they study? You must find out what their mindsets are. If you can do it regularly with enough strong feeling, eventually your mind will be- come "set." Then nothing can stop you. It is nature's law! You will reap exactly what you sow!

The former heavyweight champion, Muhammad Ali, was a master at "setting" his mind. In his early fights, he would decide in what round he wanted to knock out his opponent. Almost always, he would accomplish this unbelievable feat. So strong was his will that he would also set his opponents mind! Even before the fight, they knew that they would suddenly get "dizzy" in a certain round. . . whatever round Ali had previously decided upon! There was one fight in particular against Englishman, Henry Cooper that best showcased Ali's incredible will power and mental toughness. Ali had predicted that Cooper would be knocked out in five rounds. However, Ali himself was knocked down in the fourth round! Most people would have gotten discouraged — not Ali. He refused to let this setback hold him back. His mind remained where it had been previously set. Brother Ali got off the canvas and proceeded to whip Cooper into submission in the predicted fifth round! Ali is a living, breathing legend. He is a genius. He was a master at controlling his mind — and the minds of other people.

I must make a key point. A great part of having the ability to "set" your mind will be determined by your willingness to sacrifice long hard hours preparing yourself for eventual success. The world saw Ali beat Cooper. They saw his great stamina. They saw the quick powerful, whip like jabs. We witnessed his mind-boggling foot and hand's speed ... but the world did not see the weeks of hard training; the miles and miles of running up and down hills in heavy combat boots; the thousands of sit-ups; the rounds and rounds of sparring. Ali, no doubt, trained himself to the brink; the very edge of human capability. This training was all a great part of "setting his mind." So you must be prepared to meet with success. When your mind knows that you have done all that you can do, you will automatically be lifted up to a higher level of existence... beyond the realm of common understanding. Only the great ones have experienced this phenomenon.

Understand this truth... you cannot be stopped once your mind is permanently "set" in a given direction. Look around, the world is full of great men and women who set their minds and accomplished their lifelong goals and ambitions. Study their lives. You will discover they are not at all different from yourself. Great people are just ordinary people, with extraordinary expectations! **NATURE DICTATES THAT YOU WILL GET EXACTLY WHAT YOU FEEL YOU ARE WORTHY OF... AND YOUR FEELINGS CAN BE MEASURED BY YOUR THOUGHTS!**

Do you remember the super bowl of 1988? Doug Williams was the first Black quarterback to lead his team to a super bowl. There was Doug, pitted against what most "experts" considered to be the top-rated quarterback in the league, John Elway of the Denver Broncos.

The game started out in the worst way for Doug. With the whole world looking, Doug's team, the Washington Redskins, fell be- hind ten to nothing in the first quarter. To make matters worse, Doug slipped and badly sprained his knee! Doug's coach, Joe Gibbs, wondered about the status of his quarterback. Could he continue? Was he too seriously injured? Was he still mentally in the game?

Could Doug still lead his team? Coach Gibbs had to make a deci- sion. Gibbs pondered these questions until he looked deep into Doug's eyes. Doug had a look of complete confidence. His mind was "set" on playing, and winning! Williams reentered the game in the second quarter, badly limping, but fully determined. He went out and almost immediately threw a perfect touchdown pass. Did he stop there? No way! Doug went on to lead his team to score thirty-five second quarter points! It was the greatest performance in super bowl history! Washington won the lopsided game forty-two to ten and Doug was named the most valuable player. Understand that nothing can stop a made-up, determined, "set" mind!

Determine what you want and decide to dedicate yourself to the mission. **WELCOME OBSTACLES; THEY ARE OPPORTUNITIES TO PROVE YOUR METTLE. IF YOUR MIND IS MADE-UP OR SET, THE THINGS THAT YOU THINK ARE OBSTACLES, YOU WILL DISCOVER ARE TRULY OPPORTUNITIES IN DISGUISE. IT JUST DEPENDS ON HOW YOU CHOOSE TO VIEW THEM AND USE THEM.**

How do you set your mind? There are numerous ways. But the first thing you must do is to find out what you want. You must know where you want to go. Write down on paper a set of goals. **(As I said earlier, your mind will unquestionably pull you in any direction you "set" it on.)** Write down paragraphs detailing where you will be, what you will be doing and how you intend to do what you desire to do. Be very specific. Answer who, what, how, where and when. Also, be sure to write down what you will feel like when you reach your goals. Describe the people, setting or scenery. Let your imagination run wild! The sky is the limit! You may write either one paragraph or if the picture in your mind is clear or vivid enough, you may write five pages per goal.

Let us say that you decided to take a trip across the country. The first thing you would do is decide where you are headed. Next, you would get a map and chart a course. You would get all the items you would need for the trip. Once you have planned and prepared yourself, you are ready to proceed intelligently. You would follow your plan (the map directions). You certainly would not just go out, get in your car and start driving in any direction!

Preparation is the key! So take the time to map out your future or your destiny. Sadly, many people will map out their vacations yet fail to map out their lives! Your life is worth preparation! So go ahead and "set" your mind! And don't forget to enjoy yourself along the way. **Life should be fun! We should live our lives as if we have embarked on an exciting journey.**

So keep things in perspective. Remember not to get too caught up with certain negatives that might come your way. Even in the bleakest situation, there is always a ray of hope. You must train your mind to search for the high road. **At some point in your life, you must come to the understanding that you have to take full responsibility for your every thought, thus your every action. Your life will be whatever you think it should be!**

DESIRE

MY DESIRES ARE SUPPORTED
BY MY BELIEFS . . .
AND MY BELIEFS REFLECT
MY INNERMOST THOUGHTS.
Almas J. Sami'

5

DESIRE

The dictionary defines desire as such: "*To long or hope for; to re- quest; to invite.*" Now that is an interesting concept. Can you imagine yourself standing in front of a mirror saying, "I invite happiness into my possession!" Well, with the proper mindset, that may not be such a ridiculous idea! Some happy people would tell you that it is not always necessarily a matter of our going to get our happiness, but rather our acquiring the ability to remove mental barriers that prevent riches or happiness from finding us! This is just another way of saying that we truly do attract unto us those things and situations that reflect our innermost thoughts and feelings.

Behind this process is a tremendously powerful desire. That is a desire, not a mere wish. When you desire a thing or a happening, there is present an internal strength. You possess much stronger "feelings" for your desires than you do your wishes. But more important is the fact that wishes are more often "believed" to be unattainable. Conversely, when you really and truly have your desires in place, few obstacles can hold you back! Belief fuels de- sire. BookerT. Washington enjoyed reading the biographies of great men and women. They helped to make his own desires more believable. They were a great source of inspiration to him. Let us further explore this process of thought in an attempt to bring to light the lack of desire, lack of motivation, or feelings of inadequacy you may have experienced in the past. Perhaps we will come to know that our beliefs are connected to our desires!

Were you born in an environment with a lot of negative thinkers? We have all encountered the doom and gloom personalities who enjoy raining on everyone's parade. They get their kicks by bring- ing everybody else down to their lowly level of existence. They can turn the most pleasant of circumstances into the worst of circumstances. These people have deeply rooted hostilities, and are actually on the lookout for negative situations. I know of a young lady who is one of these "negativity seekers." Every time I am around her, she spends the whole time that we're together, arguing every good comment I make. I use to try to reform her, but I finally came to the conclusion that no matter what I did or said, she would twist it into something totally different from what I in- tended. Eventually, I got smart enough to steer clear of her altogether!

As I have said earlier, there is a reason for everything. Usually, negative thinkers are programmed to think negatively from early on in their lives. We were all born into this world with nothing but our thoughts or rather the ability to think. We arrive without money, clothing or the immediate ability to procure the basic necessities of life.

So, for the first few years of life we are dependent upon others for our welfare. There were no doubt many things you saw and de- sired between birth and the age of six. If your parents (or parent) did not have the means or the money by which to fulfill those desires, you were probably disappointed a lot of the time. It is not altogether unhealthy for a child to experience these circumstances unless he or she were made to feel undeserving of those desires.

Often parents will make a child feel guilty about wanting toys or other desires. Why? Because it relieves the guilt of not being able to supply a child with his or her wants. It is usually easier for a misunderstanding parent to face the child with anger, rather than with shame. Especially if they are barely able to supply the child with necessities! It is easy to make damaging statements like: "You are always begging for something you know you don't deserve." Not only does that child suffer for want of their desires, but now they have been told they are "undeserving." If they hear these kind of statements often enough, they began to attach their desires to their self-worth. They learn not to aim "too high." It goes without saying that most parents do not intentionally give children this faulty mindset, but the damage is done just the same.

I knew of a sister who often referred to her three year old son as a "little monkey." What are the odds of that little brother growing up with a healthy disposition? Unfortunately, there are millions of little Black boys and girls experiencing these kinds of emotional attacks. Black people often beat up one another psychologically… and unfortunately, these gruesome, mentally crippling routines usually begins in our early years when we are small, helpless and defenseless.

I cringe when I hear Black adults bragging about how they were "beaten" as youths by their parents and again by neighbors, teachers and anyone else who thought they "needed it." I tell them that those abuses go hand and hand with self-hatred, and unfortunately we pass self-hatred down from generation to generation! There is nothing to be gained from "beatings!" Or otherwise, our world would have been perfect back in the 1940s and 50s when these beatings occurred most often. Even in the face of all of the much needed "beatings", we still had problems with self-hatred,

Black on Black crime, alcohol and drug abuse… and not to mention sex abuse!

These conditions are amplified today because technology has made our world much smaller, and things happen faster and in greater measure than before. Our children are overloaded with violence… the last thing they need is violence inflected upon them by adults. They are already too violent!

Do not mistakenly believe that I am against disciplining children, however I believe that they are human beings and will learn much more from the examples set for them by the adults in their lives, rather than from being beaten. **Get your own act together, thereby giving your youth a positive role to follow and you will see the need for "beatings" decrease drastically. In other words, "STOP ABUSING OUR CHILDREN!" Teach them, show them, and most of all LOVE THEM!**

When we first enter this world, we are fresh and alive! We are full of curiosity and vitality. We are without negative thoughts or lim- its and are taught what is right or wrong by our environment. It is a natural process. Our expectations and concepts of reality are formed early on by our environmental influences. Parents are the number one influences or mind-molders.

When you were born, your parents already had a concept of what "reality" was to them. By a rather natural process, most of their feelings and thoughts found their way into your mind, thus color- ing your concepts or ideas about "reality." Desires (or the lack of desires) are often based on concepts of reality.

Let me give you a perfect example. A few years back, my wife and I decided to let our children spend the summer with their grand- parents in my hometown. I knew that this environment was very backward, at least as far as the racial climate was concerned. Al- though we had reservations, we decided to let them go on and spend their summer vacation there.

After they returned, I apologized and told them that I should have warned them about the horrible tensions between Blacks and Whites. I said I should have better "prepared" them. My oldest daughter looked at me with those big brown eyes and asked, "What racial tension?" I said, "You mean you spent two months in that place and you did not notice the racial tension?" She frowned and said, "No, we had a great time. I wish we could live there!" I was floored!

That was a typical example of how we can condition our children. We color our children's "reality" the same as our own. Had I told them about the racial tension before they left for the trip, they could have had perceived negative experiences, but because they went expecting and desiring a great time, they got exactly what they were looking for! Their desires were supported by their belief system, not mine. They got what they wanted; a fun vacation. Their parents learned a valuable lesson!

I am not implying that there was not an element of racial disharmony existing in that community, but I must believe that some of the "tension" was my own — fueled by my own experiences and faulty thinking! Their great trip could have been limited by the negative psychological baggage that I could have given them.

Forget your "limitations." Focus your attention on your hearts' truest desires. If you could hone in on those desires long and hard enough, it will become a "natural" obsession. You will then develop beliefs to support those desires. Once you have faith that those desires can become realities, your mind will simply pull you to those desires! Think of all of the great people who have managed to pull themselves up from the depths of gloom and despair by altering their thinking, thus creating an environment for positive change?

Brother El-Hajj Malik El-Shabazz, (aka Minister Malcolm X), is an excel- lent example of a person whose mind journeyed from one end of the spectrum to the other. Brother Malik used his time in prison to forge a new mind. He believed in the movement so much that he was able to change the mindset of millions of African Americans in a very short span of time.

He believed he could make a difference... the so-called Black Muslim movement was simply an avenue. His whole life was an exercise in courage, and a majestic voyage from disbelief to re- sounding belief! I am perplexed by the young brothers and sisters wearing the "X" caps and T-shirts, who know very little about the courage and belief systems of this great man. His life should be required knowledge for all of our youth.

Like Malik, you must have a burning desire to make a change. If your desire is strong enough, you will be propelled over life's rough spots. **BUT, YOU MUST HAVE A POWERFUL DESIRE, BACKED BY A POSITIVE, UPLIFTING BELIEF SYSTEM!** Few things are more heart breaking than watching the talented young brothers and sisters who get flushed down the drain because they lack the element of desire that is fortified by solid belief systems.

You have to have a burning desire for change. Change your beliefs about yourself if they are negative, self-defeating, unwanting beliefs. You have a choice in life. You can choose the low road or the high road. Everything in your life hinges on your ability to control your thinking. If you so desired, you could live your life as you dream. You must courageously take a stand and start living your life exactly the way you want. After all, it is your life. Make plans toward your desires. Plan your work and work your plan. Your desires will come true. It is a natural law!

RACISM

RACISM IS A MIRROR.
THE MORE RACIST I AM,
THE MORE RACISM IS
REFLECTED IN MY LIFE.

Almas J. Sami'

6

RACISM

African Americans have come to know racism as a fact of life. We have experienced racism on every level of our lives for all of our lives. So it is absolutely critical that we learn to deal with it properly and in a way that does not hinder or prevent us from achieving our goals.

Our mindset determines whether racism will affect us negatively, or even affect us at all! Confusion sets in when we try to deal with racism as a life principle, when in fact, it is not. Principles are always based on truths, and racism is always based on falsehoods.

We need to understand that these fanatical nuts are truly the most pathetic people that walk the face of the planet. Racism is un- godly, and is an element of hatred. Indeed racism is a product of evil in its purist form! Therefore, it is unnatural and goes against the grain of everything good and Godly. So you must understand a racist when you encounter one. Know that hatred always comes from within. It is the result of envy or jealousy.

Most Blacks do not understand that a racist actually feels inferior! Bigots feel inadequate in many areas of their lives. That is the basis of their problem. Look at the poor skinheads; small, pathetic, in- significant savages who hide behind guns. If you were to look in- side their hearts, you would find that they are full of pain and anguish. They are nothing more than worthless misfits who are resentful and frightened of other races! A person has to be twisted and hurting inside in order to hate.

People that feel love for themselves cannot help but feel love for others. **(I don't mean a false sense of love, whereby a person goes around shinning and grinning. This kind of false love reveals a person who is in search of affection.)** We can only give what we have. If we have self-love, we give love to the world. If we have self- hate, we give hatred. Through your study of human nature, you will discover that our outer world simply reflects or projects our inner world. A troubled soul simply cannot live without unrest and chaos manifesting itself in the outer world.

Put yourself in the small mind of a modern day klansman. It has become harder and harder for him to function in the manner of his ancestors of two-hundred years ago. Back then, White racists did not have to deal with Blacks on equal ground. It was easier to keep the Black man *"in his place."* They did not have to compete with their Black counterparts and could hide behind the illusion of White supremacy.

A racist never had to see his son come home from school, depressed because a little Black boy had beaten him out for the starting quarterback position on the football team. Little White fellows never had to come face to face with the notion that White is *not* superior. White men of yesteryear did not have to deal with over forty years of Black dominance in sports. They are cringing as their offspring are joining Black children in singing, "I Wanna Be Like Mike."

And we are now slowly moving into every area of human endeavor on both physical and mental plains. They surely did not have to contemplate powerful, self-determined brothers like Na'im Akbar, Maulana Karenga, Kweisi Mfume or Haki Madhubuti!

Egypt was really a land of Black Africans called Kmt... and the notion that Africans were the bringers of civilization was unthinkable. They surely did not have to deal with the new DNA discoveries that clearly shows that Black Africans were the first humans on earth... everyone came from east Africa! Today's racists cannot ignore the fact that **Jesus The Christ**, the cornerstone of Christianity, was a dark skinned, curly headed man whose mother had Ethiopian roots! By today's standard, Jesus was a Black Man!

Every year brings with it new revelations concerning African people. Over the past few decades, the White racist has steadily fallen from the contentment of his self-appointment as the only thinkers of humankind. It is much harder for them to fall from their pseudo ideals than it has been for Blacks to rise from the deplorable pits of hell on earth known as slavery! It is a long fall from the imaginary penthouse to the basement of reality. He is rapidly learning that his feelings of superiority were based on lies and misinformation. For the first time, he has come face to face with the fact that he is psychotic! He is learning that he never had the solid foundation of truth to stand upon... it is a very bitter pill to swallow.

Here he stands feeling small, inadequate and afraid. He focuses his mind on what he thinks he hates. . . anything different from his kind. He does not have the self-esteem to accept anything or any- one that is dissimilar. He does not want to acknowledge the fact consciously, that he feels badly about himself, and must therefore diligently search for and find fault in everything that differs from himself!

A bigot will spend a great deal of his time searching and looking for alibis. He must find statistics and literature that supports his distorted outlook. He will see Blacks, Hispanics, Asians, Hebrews and everyone else that is non-white as a threat. He "sees" them as a threat and becomes frightened. His fears become larger than life. He is overwhelmed. While he kneels on his hands and knees groping for reasons to continue down the pathway of hatred, he cannot help but notice bits and pieces of truth. And the simple truth is; "all of humankind is equal in the eyes of God!" The poor guy cannot go anywhere to get away from his fear and inferiority. He turns on his television; there is Tracee Ellis Ross. He turns the channel; there is Oprah Winfrey or Tony Brown. He decides to watch sports; there are tremendous athletes. He thinks Africans have taken over his country!

He cannot escape his fear. He watches the news; there are black and other persons of "color" all over the place. During the commercial, there are Japanese and Chinese products. He goes to the movies; there is Morgan Freeman, Denzel Washington, Will Smith, Chadwick Boseman or Michael B. Jordan. He reads the financial pages of the newspaper ... only to find that Koreans earn more money per capita than any other group of Americans. Everyday, he will contemplate the fact that Hispanics are the fastest growing segment in America. His self-doubt and hatred is fueled. No matter how hard he tries, he cannot escape the notion that Blacks and other people of color have "taken over."

It is a natural process of mind that he continues to focus on what is dominating his thoughts. Have you ever bought a new automobile and suddenly notice the same model or type of car on seemingly every street? Your mind lets you "see" whatever monopolizes your thoughts. You have blocked out the 250 cars that you past along the way. All you seem to notice is that particular automobile that you have been thinking about. It is natural. Well, this is the same process that our klansman friend is going through. He un- wittingly ignores the strides of his White brethren. For all he can focus on are the advances of so-called "minorities." It literally drives him mad. His fears are greatly amplified or exaggerated in his feeble mind.

The poor guy cannot walk down the street with his wife and pass a sharp, good-looking brother without feeling sexually inadequate. He secretly thinks his wife would like nothing more than a night at home with that "Big Black Stud." She has to try and prove to him that she is not turned on by the brother in the car next to them at the stop light, or at the checkout stand or in the mall.

He is consumed with the notion that he is inadequate in ways that Black men are powerful and potent. He cannot help thinking these thoughts because he has bought into all of the myths. His whole life has become a lie. He has become a sad, miserable wimp of a man who is trapped in the self-contained prison of his own mind. Fear is at every turn. His anger and hatred towards himself grows. It is critical for us to understand this breed and "see" them for what they truly are… frightened White people! Do not let these wretched little people rain on your parade! Do not even stop to give them the time of day. We spend far too much time dwelling upon what these people think and do. Let them write their little "bell-curve" books and pretend that they are "*intelligent.*" They have a right to their opinions… no matter how misguided and twisted they may be.

However, most White racists are not of the skinhead or klansman variety. Most are average people who are not even aware that they are racist. They get very angry when we accuse them of being bigots because they know that they do not harbor *conscious* ill feelings toward Blacks. However there are two main reasons that they *should* feel superior to

Blacks. First is an educational system that elevates Whites to the level of virtual gods. They learn early in school that White males did everything! They broke through with every medical breakthrough. Climbed every mountain. Settled every settlement. Invented every invention. Tamed a "dark" and wild world.

Although Whites do possess an impressive record of achievement over the past five hundred years, our history books are replete with story after story where White males are depicted as the *only* people to achieve. Other races (and the female gender) are either virtually omitted, or have had their inventions "white washed." **We learn that all of the sciences were born of White male minds. When it became obvious that Black men and women from KMT, Alkebu-lan (Egypt, Africa) were responsible for the foundations of medical science and mathematics etc., they either do not mention it, or claim that these Africans were dark skinned, kinky haired WHITE PEOPLE!**

White extremists in academia and the media have gone to extraordinary lengths to keep history as white and as "pure as the driven snow." This indoctrination at our schools and over the air waves has created a society full of Whites who believe to the very core of their being that they are superior or that they hold a monopoly on truth. That is what happens when only one side of any story is told. The OJ Simpson criminal and civil trials are perfect examples of what happens when the manipulators control and direct the thinking of an unsuspecting people. Anyone who saw the criminal trial on television got twice as much information that pointed to Simpson's innocence that those who had to rely on the White American media.

The media simply over reported the evidence against Simpson, and grossly under reported or neglected altogether to report the evidence that pointed towards his innocence.

A great number of Whites believed Simpson to be innocent judging by the massive number of Whites who cheered him on his journey home from jail. But the media kept reporting that Blacks and Whites are simply diametrically opposed. As time went on, more and more Whites were *conditioned* by a carefully crafted plan to make them believe that Simpson was guilty.

That is exactly how the masses are controlled by those who are the shapers of thought! Further, this is why you see so many Whites who are racists on levels that they are not even aware of themselves. They simply feel superior on a gut level... it is by design. It is unconscious! In their conscious minds a racist is a klansman who hates Blacks and simply would not tolerate our presence in this country. Not many Whites fall into that category.

They see themselves as open-minded, understanding people who will *"give"* Blacks their due. *"Why I have had lots of Black friends."* They will give you a tale of a *"wonderful Black"* whom they genuinely have deep affection for, and they believe that they simply could not have those feelings if they were racists. They overlook the fact that they think this wonderful Black was *"different from most Blacks you see."* These matters are far too deep for the masses to consciously rest upon, for our world is shallow and most minds (Black or White) do not have the training to look beneath the surface to the core of matters. Understand these truths when dealing with Whites in America and you will be able to free yourself of your own hostile notions and frustrations. Understanding will alleviate your pain and your anger for Whites will soon dissipate.

This faulty educational system leaves Africans feeling inferior on the same deep, sub level of unconsciousness. **(Learn your own ancestor's version of history and you will no longer be held hostage to White academic superiority!)**

In fighting his unconscious "feelings" of inferiority the Black racist becomes angry, bitter and bigoted himself. He will magnify insignificant racial incidences in his inferior mind and find phantom racism where racism does not exist. He looks at the mountain of white superiority evidence placed before him by the educational system and concludes in his ignorance of his own true and accurate history that Whites are evil and wicked... "that accounts for White folks' success" he tells himself. He foolishly concludes that Whites accomplished their feats only by way of trickery or at the expense of other races.

Second of the major reasons that Whites *should* feel superior to Blacks is due to our very own actions. We wear their names, adore their light skin and straight hair and if that is not enough, we will serve them, buy from them and trust their judgment long before we would another Black person. As long as African people the world over honor White males by clinging to their surnames; and so long as Africans continue to consider White looks as "ideal" (i.e. straightened hair, light skin etc.), we will continue to be viewed as second rate. Simply because we view ourselves as second rate. A free thinking and sensible people simply would not hold others up higher than themselves. If you doubt the importance of these mental errors or if you do not consider them to be injurious to the African psyche, then I challenge you to find ninety percent of White males who wear African surnames. Or eighty-five percent of White women fashioning Afro's, braids, or dreadlocks. Or ninety- nine percent of Whites who know more about African History that European History. The bottom line is that most Whites see themselves as the best, and unfortunately, we agree with them.

There have been notions among some of our leaders that Blacks cannot be racist because we do not have enough power to affect a negative change in White folks lives. While that may by true, I do not understand how one could deny the obvious. A rock is a rock, whether it is the size of a dime or a two-ton bolder. We miss the point when we spend time playing with words. The judgment that must be arrived at is that a racist is a small and embittered person who harbors deeply rooted tensions and anxieties. Yet that person is afraid to look inwardly for the solutions and answers to life's questions as they pertain to her own growth and development. A racist must deal inwardly with herself and address her own self hatred, whether they be White or Black.

A Black racist is also trapped in his self-made, self-contained mental stockade. He thinks that the "White man" or "the man" is out to hold him back. He ignores "the Oprah Winfreys, Tyler Perrys and Chadwick Bosemans". He cannot follow their examples of success because he does not believe in himself. He does not believe he has the potential to rise above the "White man." He too will buy into the many myths and lies and use them to direct his life. It does not matter how many successful African Americans cross his path, he will be blind to their accomplishments because he is too busy searching for reasons to justify his inadequacies.

Deep down inside he wishes he were a White man. He believes he would have to be White in order to live a truly happy life. These are not necessarily conscious thoughts or inferiority's, but his feelings will not betray him. He does not have a clue as to why his life is such a failure. If he would seek counsel in the depths of his soul, he would quickly come to the realization that he is his own worst enemy. He was born with all of the tools needed to put his life in order, yet he will curse others outwardly and defy himself inwardly.

Unknowingly, he is a kindred spirit of the White racist. He has a list of "statistics" and "stories" that he believes will support his pitiful racist mentality. However, he cannot escape the myths that go against him. He truly thinks

Whites are born smarter than Blacks. He is secretly attracted to blonde hair and blue-eyed women because he believes he is elevated when he is with them. **(A Black marrying a White out of true love is altogether different. From a male standpoint, interracial crossing is usually reflective of just how inferior Black and White racists truly are. The average Black will go with White women because in his mind, he is showing the White male that he is his equal. He has captured the "Whitemans" prize possession ... the White woman! Again, remember that his aim is to be like or mimic the White male. {Man, he is squatting in tall cotton now!} Meanwhile, the inferior White male will often seek to bed a Black woman, because in doing so, he is being elevated for having pleased the "Blackmans" woman! To his warped way of thinking, the Black man is seen as the man of all men ... and if he can actually please the "Blackmans" woman, then he is indeed christened ... A MAN}** Insanity is the cornerstone of racism; Stupidity is its very foundation!)

Moreover, a Black racist will curse every White person in existence and in the next breath, he will call his brother a "nigga!" Deep within the psyche of brothers and sisters who outwardly claim to hate Whites lie the seed of self-hatred. Resentment and jealousy are by-products of an unrested, uncultivated, unloved soul! This self-hatred continues until the pain and negative feelings are properly dealt with. No amount of boasting about how evil and sinister the "White man" is will alleviate the pain of self-hatred! The road to wellness and happiness begins within! Someone once said that the longest journey is the one that starts on one side of your head and ends on the other! Forget about focusing on White people. If you feel hatred towards others, it is an absolute that you are merely reflecting the feelings of self-hatred that are lying dormant within the crevices of your being!

Often the most resentful Blacks are the last ones to embrace African values or study African histories. They will curse the White man, yet refuse to rid themselves of a White slave master's name. They will curse the White woman even while burning their scalp attempting to make their hair look like their White "enemy." I have always been amazed by the fact that a brother could claim to hate the so-called "White devil" and then turn right around and give his son a European name and continue the heritage and remnants of slavery!

Their true problem is that they are jealous and resentful. They would be surprised to find that a healthy knowledge of themselves and their heritage would alleviate much of their pain. We must come to the conclusion that humans are neither above or below one another in stature as far as nature is concerned. Racial hatred is a man-made disease. If you will rid yourself of your own slave mentality, you will no longer be a slave to racism or to racists. You are always free to choose your thoughts. Get started molding your world from within your own mind and heart... The world without will follow suit.

Now, there is another type of racist within the African community. Their hatred for themselves and for other Blacks run the deepest. It is the racist who bitterly hates his own kind. They hate the fact that they were born African. They especially hate poor Blacks that embarrass them in front of their White buddies. Most of these racist brothers and sisters are "educated" and tend to have nice jobs and live in "nice" neighborhoods.

They continually run from the things in life that reminds them that they are African. To their warped minds, a big house and a fat paycheck makes them equal to Whites. Their driving aim in life is to be accepted by their White chums. The more they are like White people, the happier these pitiful brothers and sisters are. They are in fact, cheap, meager replicas of Whites... *synthetic* White people, if you will. It is sad because these are the very people who could be of great help in elevating less fortunate Blacks. On every street in every "ghetto" there is at least one person who is in the frame of mind to be helped if these "sophisticated" brothers and sisters would but lend a hand or offer a few words of encouragement. If we all were united for a common cause we could uplift ourselves rather than depend on so many government programs to do what can only be accomplished by us individually and collectively.

I first began taking notes on these miseducated Blacks when I began doing research for this book. I wanted to rap to "successful" brothers and sisters in order to tap their resources. My idea was to retrieve their principles of success in order to pass them on to my readership. To my surprise, I came across more snobbery among these types than among their White counterparts whom they are so busy trying to emulate! I found more often than not that they would be more inclined to give me acceptance when I dressed in a three-piece suit. On those days when I wore jeans and a sweat shirt, they would not give me the time of day. They shunned me in a way that I will not soon forget. Their disdain for me was piercing. Their disgust rivaled the reddest of rednecks. I am careful not to throw them all in a negative category, but the fact remains I encountered hostilities all too often.

In retrospect, I have to chuckle because they reminded me of the character, "Sarge" in the movie, "A Soldiers Story." Good ole Sarge did all he could to be accepted by Whites. In his pursuit he ended up literally killing other brothers who did not meet with White folks approval. Even though he could not be White, he would have happily settled for second best— to at least be accepted by Whites. To be a crude imitation of Whites was indeed a worthy ambition. And the final analysis showed that he was psychologically drained and crushed at discovering that no matter how much he placated, and tried to snuggle up to his *superiors*, Whites still would not accept him as their equal. So I say to these Black racists; loosen your ties, raise your proud heads and decide to dedicate yourselves to helping your hurting brothers and sisters. You may be surprised to find that those so-called "*uneducated*" tribesmen and women may teach you a thing or two.

A few years ago, while in San Francisco on business, I had the pleasure of spending the day with a "wino." I stood on the corner with this brother and took in his knowledge and experiences. He was so overwhelmingly keen that I quickly realized that his mental capabilities and understanding far surpassed many of the "educated" or "professional" Blacks that I had been interviewing. It would be truly inspirational to our youth if we could somehow get the knowledge from our street people and pass it on for the betterment of our youth. We have too much brain power lying around not benefiting any of us.

Now the most sinister Black racist is the one who hides his or her own inferiority behind the cloak of Black history, or Afrocentricity. Like the Klansman, they will have all of the *"research"* to prove that Whites are inherently evil. They believe that Blacks are the children of God, and by *"nature"* are inherently good, and Whites are children of the devil, or that their *"nature"* is somehow aligned with that of Satan. Every vice, malady or behavioral problem that we suffer will find it's root at the foot of that dastardly "Whiteman!" They unmindfully make the "Whiteman" all knowing and all powerful and as a result, consign our responsibility *and* our power to White human beings.

NOTHING HAPPENED TO US WITHOUT OUR ASSISTANCE! We were a divided and tribalized people long before the arrival of the European and White Arab poachers.

Tribe fought tribe, stole tribe, sold tribe and ultimately tribe killed tribe! The institution of slavery would never have lasted had it not been for Black "House-slaves" allowing themselves to become tools of the White slave master. The weak will seek out the strong for nourishment... even if that *"nourishment"* is only a figment of their improperly cultivated imagination! **We must learn that if there is to be a perpetual abuser, there must by natural law be a perpetually compliant and willing victim.**

We must quest to remedy our own weaknesses as a race if we are to move on to higher ground. Whites, Asians, native Americans and every other people on this earth must remedy their own ills first. In his timeless and masterful book, **"The Mis-Education of the Negro," Dr. Carter G. Woodson said it best when he wrote, "The differentness of races, moreover, is no evidence of superiority or of inferiority. This merely indicates that each race has certain gifts which the others do not possess. It is by the development of these gifts that every race must justify its right to exist."**

The real tragedy is that many of these hostile and wrathful Afrocentric brothers and sisters could be of great use as instructors, motivators and leaders of our communities, yet they turn people off with their animosity, bitterness and contempt for other races. They tend to live and dwell in a negative world, which is merely reflective of their pessimistic and crippling thinking. **If you do not know that all living forms are an integral part of this magnificent affair called life; then you my friends are thought- shackled in the worse way! The same life force that flows within White people is made up of the same "stuff" that makes us all breathe... the life force does not discriminate; but trifling, and backwards thinking humans do! The problem with this world is that we do not "know" that we are intrinsically the same!**

No my brothers and sisters, Black history should bring us closer to each other *and* closer to other races, or at least leave you with a better understanding of life from every angle. **If God saw fit to create this world, the least you could do is cherish divine conception; in all shapes, sizes and colors, less your mind be shackled!**

FAITH

MY FAITH IS UNSEEN BY ALL . . .
EXCEPT MY HEART'S EYE.
IN THERE, WITHIN THE DARK
RHYTHMIC PULSING, I FIND MY STRENGTH
WHICH IS FORTIFIED BY MY VISION

Almas J. Sami'

7

FAITH

Most people do not understand the absolute power of faith. Faith is actually a gift! Fortunate is the one who climbs to this lofty realm of consciousness. We can realize faith by repeating over and over in our mind, thoughts that suggest we will get what we want or desire.

Muhammad Ali would constantly repeat his boxing predictions. Many people felt Ali was a prophet. Others thought the fights were rigged because more often than not Ali would be correct. If he said he would win in six rounds, he won in six rounds! How could Ali do that? Well, he did it by utilizing natural thought laws. He repeated over and over what he desired. The more he repeated the words, the more faith he built up in his mind and heart. Soon, everyone within shouting distance began building faith in his predictions. Does that mean Ali merely spouted off at the mouth? Hardly, for he first had a desire to win at a certain point in the fight. He then laid plans for the fight or trained for the fight. All the while he trained, he expressed or suggested to himself the idea that he would fulfill his desire. The rest is boxing history. You have probably heard the statement, "faith moves mountains." Faith can also thrust you upward to your loftiest pinnacle!

One of the most moving stories I have ever encountered was that of a brother named Emmitt Jackson. One fatal night, someone set his next door neighbors' apartment on fire. The flames spread throughout the entire complex and as a result, Jackson was burned on over 80 percent of his body. He lost his eyelids, ears, lips, nose, one of his eyes and half of both arms. It was not until six months later, while still on his back in the hospital living in searing pain did he learn that his wife and daughter had died in the fire. His emotional and physical pain was beyond imagination. Yet through all of this, Jackson remained a tower of strength! He is an inspiration to thousands of hurting people who have heard his story.

Jackson has managed to make it through all of his misfortune by maintaining an unwavering faith in God, and in himself. Jackson uses the principles of faith every minute of every hour in everyday of his life! Today, he stands tall; a living testament to the fundamental laws governing faith. So what about you, my friend? Will you resolve to utilize even a fraction of the faith that Jackson uses every moment of his life? Faith is an emotion. A very powerful emotion. It is a power that goes right to the very core of your being. In other words, you will "feel" faith. The deeper the "feelings", the closer you are to the thing or situation that you desire.

If you were to plant a flower; water and nurture it daily, the flower will soon grow and sprout and thus become a reality. It is likewise with your desires. Plant them, [or plan them] and water them daily, [or write and confess aloud] with conviction. In the case of the flower, the chemical reactions with water and sun will produce a result... growth. With your desires, writing and stating them aloud will also create a cosmic chemical reaction. Faith is that chemical reaction. Just as the flower blossoms, so will your wildest dreams.

When you think positive thoughts, developing faith will be easier. You will see that the common thread throughout this book is the importance of a proper mindset, or the ability to channel thoughts. Thinking is the true business in life. Thinkers rule the world, they always have, and they always will. It is a natural law!

Look to our religions for great testimonies of faith. For **Jesus** told Peter in the Book of Mark, chapter 11 to, **"Have faith in God. Verily I say unto you, whosoever shall say unto this mountain, be thou taken up and cast into the sea; and shall not doubt in his heart, but shall believe that what he saith cometh to pass; he shall have it. Therefore I say unto you all things whatsoever ye pray and ask for, believe that ye receive them and ye shall have them."** Those are pretty words, but let us take a closer look. What are the operative or key words used? Let us break them down. First of all He said have faith in God. Right away He lets you know that this is a divine principle ... a natural law. Secondly, He gave instruction to "say" unto this mountain. In other words, you must speak out loud the results you seek or want to accomplish! He said , "All things whatsoever ye pray for, ask for." What is a prayer? Words "spoken" to God.

Next, He said, "Believe that ye receive them, and ye shall have them." He did not say to believe you are"going" to receive. But rather He said to believe that you have already received, or believe that your desires have "cometh to pass." In other words, you should have the mindset that you already have the thing you desire. The great boxer Evander Holyfield went into his battle with Mike Tyson a decided underdog. All of the "experts" said that Tyson would walk right through him. They in fact questioned whether Holyfield would come out of the fight alive! But Evander had an absolute consuming faith in God and in his own resolve. He, in fact guaranteed a win before the fight! History has now recorded that magnificent battle in which Evander Holyfield dismantled Mike Tyson and showed the world that faith is indeed creator of reality!

It is always easy to identify a man or woman of faith. They have a presence or a mindset that suggest supreme confidence. It is impossible to have confidence without faith. **The Prophet Muhammad**, had many trying moments before His message was accepted. He was laughed at, humiliated and even stoned, yet He went into the quiet of His heart and continued to build faith. Today there are over a billion faithful Muslims who testify to the Prophets' convictions. {His life and times are brilliantly chronicled in a must read book titled: **"WELCOME TO ISLAM" By Doctor Khalid Abdullah Tariq Al-Mansour.**} Incidentally, many of the slaves from the Motherland who came to this country were Muslims. So it is safe to say that we should pay at the very least a passing interest in this magnificent faith — as well as other spirit touching belief systems from your ancient **ALKEBU-LAN** fore parents. Our world is thousands and thousands of years old ... explore it!

So build your faith, express your aims, desires and goals. Be sure to express them in the positive. In other words, "say it like you al- ready have it!" Give thanks before you get it! Picture how you would feel if your goals were already at hand. In the passages of your mind, there is no difference between fact and fiction. We have the ability to create reality and shape our lives in whatever fashion that our minds deem to be "fact." Express yourself, to your- self!

For instance, if your goal is to get a new car, picture exactly how the car looks. What kind of car is it? What color is the exterior and interior? Go to the lot and test drive your car. Be sure and get some brochures. Picture yourself driving it. Where will you drive it; to work, to school, to the supermarket or the business meetings? Picture what your car would look like parked in your garage or in front of your house. Who else will ride in the car? Can you hear your favorite music playing on the stereo? What does the car smell like? How do you feel as you drive down the street? What does the engine look like? What will you put in the trunk? Are you going to pay cash for it? If not, what will your down payment be? Will you trade your present car in; if so, see yourself driving the old car in picking up your new car. You must also form in your mind the means by which you will earn money for the car. You must actually see yourself doing the things that will make enough money for the purchase of the car.

Look again at the above example of how to set goals. When picturing, be sure to use all five of your senses. You will note that I have involved more than one of our senses. I used sight, smell, touch and just as important, I tapped "feelings."

You have to create vivid pictures of your desires in your minds' eye. With a clear picture in your mind, you will then began to actually "feel" your desires better. Your brain is like a television. You can react to the pictures and images in your mind by using the same principle that advertisers utilize when they get you to run out and buy their products!

For instance, it is no secret that beer companies target young men. Their marketing efforts are aimed primarily at the young, male viewer. And how do they get their attention? By showing scantily clad women in bathing suits just waiting to have fun with any nut with a beer in his hands! Knowing that sex is a high priority among average young men, they can create the image of people having the time of their lives ... as long as they are gulping down the right brand of beer.

In other words, the pictures that they conjure up will tap very strong emotions of the young viewer; after-all, sex is a very powerful emotion that most young men are readily in touch with. So the next time the little guy goes in for a beer, he will remember the commercial, feel the same emotions that he felt when he watched the commercial and automatically reach for that particular brand of beer. The fact that beer makers spend billions of dollars annually on such commercials lends testimony that this concept works!

You must "play up" the pictures and images of your desires in your mind, utilizing those same emotional appeals that advertisers use. Remember; the clearer the picture, the more exciting the picture, the more emotion that you can tap, the closer you are to your goals and dreams. Most people either do not have a mental picture of their goals or if they do, it is not a clear, concise image for their mind to see and use.

UTILIZE ALL OF YOUR BRAIN! You must actually see your dreams, goals, and desires in your minds' eye. You must feel your dreams, goals and desires in your heart. After you have written your narrative paragraphs, record them on an audio cassette. Then everyday, close your eyes and listen to it. If you have written them correctly, you will be able to actually see the pictures that your voice conjures up as you listen.

Spend some time everyday going over and over your goals. Just like Muhammad Ali, build faith by repetition. Go over it again and again until it becomes a reality in your mind. You will build faith. Your mind will begin to pull your dreams to you! When you have faith, you are well on your way to your targeted destination. Faith is the fuel that makes your dreams grow into reality. Without faith, all is lost, but with faith, all is possible!

SUCCESS

I LIVE NOT FOR A MILLION
DOLLAR HOME, BUT RATHER A
MILLION DOLLAR MIND!
I LIVE FOR SUCCESS YEARLY, MONTHLY, WEEKLY,
DAILY, HOURLY AND YES, MINUTE BY MINUTE.
I KNOW THAT SUCCESS
IS NOT THE END OF A PROCESS,
BUT RATHER
THE PROCESS ITSELF.

Almas J. Sami'

8

SUCCESS

To succeed means to achieve or to reach a desired result; to positively bring to a close. Really, success can mean different things to different people. One man's success can be another woman's failure or vice versa.

Ultimately, like everything else I have talked about so far, to succeed or to fail hinges on one thing... the mindset or thinking pattern of the individual. If a person decided to think his or her way towards a goal, success is guaranteed.

Berry Gordy, the great mind behind the Motown empire also came from humble beginnings. He saw that there was not a record company that adequately harnessed and showcased Black talent. **(When you learn to think on a higher plain, your mind lets you "see" or "notice" things and situations that are only visible to one whose mind is on a certain lofty level.)** He sat out to cultivate African talent and serve the Black public. Gordy not only served the Black public, but he went on to revolutionize the entire music industry!

A great number of successful African Americans made it big by finding a way to serve other African Americans. Tony Brown, Sharazhad Ali, John Johnson, Marva Collins, Maulana Karenga, and Tyler Perry to name but a few genius trail blazers who sought to offer great services to the Black public.

(Black Entertainment Television). Dr. Jawanza Kunjufu is well on his way to redefining education. Even Muhammad Ali went to another level after he embraced his Blackness. I am not saying that we should seek to serve "only" Black people, but if you are searching for a way to succeed, then you should take the lead from the many Great Black Geniuses and look to serve your people first. Just look around you, there are a host of things that you can offer African Americans!

A very important element of success is having the ability to take setbacks without loosing your footing; without loosing hope and without giving up on your goals. There are sure to be times when things do not go exactly the way you might have planned. If you utilize setbacks; if you put them in their proper place, you will find that they actually help you. They give guidance.

It is like driving a car to a certain destination. You may have planned a route and may be following the road you mapped out, but all of a sudden you run into a detour sign. Do you give up on the trip altogether? Of course not... because your mind is set on going in that direction. And if you examined the conditions, you would see that the detour sign has an arrow pointing you in the right direction — telling you where you must go in order to reach your destination!

Sure, you may be a little inconvenienced, but if you would stop to think about it, the detour may save you from danger. The bridge may be out further down the road! Or the road may be in such bad condition that you would ruin your car if you drove over it! The obstacle is really there to aid and assist you! So now you see, after examining the setback or detour, you were really given instructions to "ensure" your safe arrival to your destination. If your goal is a worthy ambition, then it is worth putting up with all of the downfalls and inconveniences along the way. You are assured of success if you will take the time to learn how to read the signs of life. You will learn to accept and even be thankful for the detours of life.

I am sure that Brother Lewis Latimer ran into thousands of de- tours while he was inventing the first electric lamp. After "thousands" of failures, most people would have gotten discouraged and "quit." But Lewis got more and more motivated and inspired after each setback or failure. Why? Because with each failure, he realized he was just that much closer to success! He now knew another path or roadway that he should not travel down. He simply read the detour signs for what they were ... directions and instructions on where to go from that given point in the project! He "thought" failures were actually guideposts! What a tremendous example of how our minds are to be used. Lewis Latimer also improved Thomas Edisons' invention of the light bulb by making them last longer. Additionally, he drew the designs for Alexander Bell's tele- phone patent! Were it not for Latimer's keen mind, we might not see at night or communicate as we do today. He was a master thinker!

Another key to achieving success is knowing what you want. What is your desire? What would you like to accomplish? Search and research until you find out what you are all about. You may find that you are capable of or have a desire to do more than any single endeavor.

Look at Venus and Serena Williams. They excelled after receiving instruction from their great father, Richard Williams Jr who was a self taught teacher of tennis. He decided that he would teach his two fantastic daughters while living in Compton, CA. There weren't many tennis instructors in the area, so he taught them himself after studying tennis in books and magazines. If you are looking for a parenting role model, I would google the story of Richard Williams Jr and his two incredible daughters! He revolutionized the game of tennis.

It is critical that you know what you want and have faith in your ability to succeed. **THERE IS SIMPLY NO WAY TO STOP A MADE-UP MIND! It is also critical that you know "why" you want what you want. Anyone can do anything if they give themselves enough reasons. Knowing "why" you are in want of your goals is very important.**

Spike Lee, the great movie director, said he did not want to succeed because of money or fame or any of the like. He simply loves doing what he does. This is a very powerful point. The reward then comes from the very act or endeavor itself.

Sit down and write a list of what you want or aspire to do. Next, make a list of why you want to succeed at reaching your goal. Then write why you think you will succeed. Write a narrative or a few paragraphs detailing what, why and how you intend to reach your aims or your goals. Be very clear about it. The more detailed and clear you are in writing this narrative, the more "set" your mind will be. In other words, you will have a defined, definite picture for your mind to follow. You will have a map!

Also, be sure that you know what success means to you. You could ask one-hundred people what success means to them, and you would probably get one-hundred different answers. But let me tell you my definition of true success: When you can wake up in the morning, and sing with the birds; when you can bask in the warmth of the sun; when you can sit and marvel at the power of an afternoon thundershower, and be at one with that power; when you can look deep into the eyes of a loved one, and can transmit that love back to them; when you can look at that

Black face in the mirror and thank God, you my friend have arrived. Success and you are one. Understand that no amount of money, or material possession will bring you more success than love… awareness of the need to give and receive love will render you more success than you can handle!

MYTHS . . . BREAKING BARRIERS

I LIVE UNAFFECTED BY MYTHS,
FOR I CHOOSE NOT TO TREAD UPON
MURKY WATERS WHERE SWIMS
THE COMMON MIND.

Almas J. Sami'

9

MYTHS . . . BREAKIN BARRIERS

Do you believe in any of the many myths and superstitions that we have heard all of our lies? I once had a White friend whose grandfather taught him that Blacks are not as smart as Whites because our skulls were three or four times thicker than Whites; thus there was not sufficient room for a brain the size of a White man's! The poor old man went to his grave misinformed — clinging on to myths. Had this old fellow been schooled in the true history of humankind, he would have known that the group of people with the largest brains, belonged to that of the "Bush-man," a tribe in southern Africa!

I once knew a very "liberal" White girl, a second year medical student, who believed the same myth. I asked her why she believed it, and she said, "I don't know why." The funny thing is, she was dating a Black man at the time! Perhaps she considered him to be her big Black buck! Negative myths about Blacks are so in- grained in many White peoples' minds that they are almost unaware of their own thoughts and certainly do not have a clue as to why they think and feel the way they do.

At work one day I asked a White colleague why he was racist. He looked puzzled, and even hurt when he asked, "Jamil, how could you say such a thing, when you know how much I like and admire you?" Quickly, before he began to cry, I asked what he knew of African history. He said he knew quite a bit, and started to rattle off the names of Martin Luther King Jr., Booker T. Washington, Frederick Douglass and other prominent African Americans.

I asked him what he knew of our history prior to slavery… to which he said, "There wasn't much African history prior to the Slave Trade." I followed up with a simple question; 'How can you not be a racist if you believe we were completely insignificant prior to mingling with Whites? Can you not see that within the deepest fibers of your being, you believe that nearly everything of significance came about by way of the White race? You believe that the Son of God is White, indeed, God is White! You believe that Whites developed the world, indeed civilized the world. You believe all of the math and sciences were products of White minds… in short, you believe the White race to be the front runners in practically every human endeavor, save music and athletics!'

I began to tell him my version of the histories of the world, a view that is inclusive of every race known to humankind! Needless to say, he had a hard time coming to grips with much of what I was telling him.

The last question I asked him was; "Have you ever read the history of Africa as related by Africans?" After he said no, there was only one other question to ask… "How can you possibly get an accurate history of the continent when you have yet to read the teachings of any of Africa's' scholars?" The obvious answer as far as he was concerned was, "I did not know that there were African Scholars" ... which brought us back to my original statement regarding his racist outlook.

It is unfortunate that his ancestors set him up in this unreal, pseudo "White is right" world. There are millions of demented White people who are having a tough time coming to grips with the realization that they are not a "special" or "chosen" people! As more and more correct information and history is revealed, they are having to climb down from their "make-believe" world of White supremacy.

One of the more common misconceptions is that we are a race of "Negro" or "Negroid" people. It never occurred to our ancestors who were enslaved to question the terms. They were of a mindset to accept almost everything that their former masters handed down to them ... including their names! Think about this; White slave masters' named one of three "possessions". They named their wives, their children and their pets. Where do you suppose their slaves fell in this hierarchy? Perhaps somewhere between children and pets! And often, they were placed below the level of the beast ... even if the filthy master fathered the slaves, he would still view them as sub-human! In order to "season" a person to become a "good" slave, they had to be taught to give up a very important human trait ... the power to define one's self. Along with the defining of one's self comes the ability to define goals and avenues. A sense of confidence is then cultivated, allowing one to dream of a better day, a brighter future. And more importantly, it ensures that one will take action towards those expectations.

The time has come for us to accept the challenge and responsibilities of becoming self-thinking, self-loving people. Our more re- cent ancestors of 130 years ago did not have the choices that we have today. They knew not "from whence they came!" However, the fact that we are here today lends testimony to their strength, courage and determination. Those who managed to keep their wits about them dreamed of a day when we would be "whole" again! We do not have to face the hardships and obstacles that they en- countered.

For the most part, the yoke of bygone atrocities and abuses have been lifted. The price of which was paid in full by the blood of our marvelous ancestors. So we must rethink ourselves, and reshape our futures... and begin to question the wisdom of calling ourselves "nigga" and "negro." We must cease the practice of handing our children surnames which were given to us in the same fashion that one would give a dog a bone! We must rid ourselves of the habit of looking to others for the solutions to our problems. The days of holding hands and singing "We Shall Overcome" have long past... unless we collectively sing, "We Shall Overcome — OURSELVES!"

When our ancient African ancestors walked the face of this earth, they built new worlds, forged new avenues of thought. They settled, they conquered, they ushered civilization into Europe, Asia and the rest of the world! And yet, here we stoop; the descendants of kings and queens and earth shakers, thinking and believing that we should be someone other than whom we are... it's MADNESS!

We do not have a vision. We will not have vision until we began to take the wheels of our minds and map out our own destinies. We seek the comfort of drugs to avoid this responsibility. I am not only talking about alcohol and cocaine and the like, but also the drugs that make us sleepwalk through life. Such drugs as going to church and just handing all of our problems over to **Jesus**. These were not the character traits of **Jesus**. (Yeshua Ben Yusef), He was an action person. It is true that he relied on the power of God. He allowed himself to become a vessel for that power.

He tapped that magnificent power "while" he worked to make this a better world. He did not lie down like a sheep and just "go with the tide." He was a thinking man! No one defined him. He defined himself and his mission! Such was the legacy that he left us. He showed how we can achieve by optimizing the power of thought. He showed us that our minds are actual instruments to be utilized each and every day. He would not approve of us shirking our responsibilities to ourselves, our children, our communities or our lives!

If we would make self-examination a priority, we would find the solutions to our problems. We would know how to take our children off the streets. We would provide them with leadership. Most African Americans will preach about how hard life is for Black people. Well, life will surely seem hard to a people who have yet to grasp the fundamentals of human understanding and self-knowledge.

We must come to know that the remedies for our ills must be fashioned in our minds! The sooner we grasp this simple truth, the sooner we will began to really address our concerns about poverty, crime, gang violence and the like. We would come to understand that self-hatred is the primary obstacle to understanding our humanism. When we grasp the intricacies of our humanity, we will then be equipped to deal with this world! Even so called, "wild animals" know and understand themselves. Dogs know dogs, cats know cats, lions know lions, yet we do not know the basics of who we are or the elementary functions of our human capacity. All is possible, but unfortunately we keep close company with myths given to us by other people.

It is sad enough that we should allow lies and myths from others to hinder us. But it is far more devastating for us to believe in the many myths and lies that we keep company with regarding ourselves! Often myths regarding our own competence will keep us from trusting each other, depending on each other, indeed placing our lives in each others hands. We indeed have all of the brain power in place to get our own house in order if we would but believe in each other, then resolve to fully serve one another. Earlier in life I discovered that one of the hardest things to do was to give Blacks the same level of professionalism that I had given Whites. I would foolishly go all out when serving Whites, yet when I ran across Blacks, I found myself slacking and easing up. Partly because I did not believe Blacks would appreciate excellence, nor did we deserve it. I bought into the myth that we are sub-human beings who did not quite measure up to Whites. We need to establish our own standards in life, both as individuals and as a collective. Go on about your business at hand; turn a deaf ear to myths. You do not need to carry that excess baggage around in your mind. And while you are dumping your own mental garbage, lend a helping hand to your confused, distrustful and disrespected brothers and sisters. One of the myths about us is that we are as crabs in a bucket; as soon as one reaches the top, the others will grab a hold of him and pull him back down. Let's turn that around. Make yourself so mighty that you will be strong enough to uplift those who are grabbing a hold of your coat tail! Give them a piggyback ride to glory! Seek truths and you will not be affected or hindered by propaganda placed before you by others who deem themselves your enemy. If we had a mind to, we could wipe hundreds of years of confusion and misunderstanding within the short span of one generation. However, nothing will change for us until we collectively come to the understanding that we have the power to affect such change. The power to change has always been within our grasp... but we must make the effort. Personally, with conviction, you can renew your mind and myths will fall from your consciousness, thus leaving room to fill your mind with keys to internal personal power.

DIRECTION

I CHART MY COURSE . . .
FOR I KNOW THAT THERE ARE MANY
WHO STAND READY AND WILLING
TO DIRECT THOSE WHO CHOOSE
NOT TO DIRECT THEMSELVES.

Almas J. Sami'

10

DIRECTION

Life is full of ups and downs. It is very important for you to be able to deal with down periods. Most of us can deal with life much more effectively when things are going great. Everything is wonderful when everything is wonderful! But how many of us can deal effectively when wonderful turns horrible? A great person once said that the measure of a man or woman can only be assessed when they are thrust into the jaws of calamity, heartbreak or despair.

Many people will get "down" when things do not go according to plan. It is natural to feel a bit discouraged when you experience setbacks or heartaches. But you should always be able to bring yourself out of these small bouts of depression. It may not always be easy, but it is a very simple process of thought.

Whenever you get depressed, it is because of the thoughts you are carrying. You are focusing on negative or depressing thoughts. The longer you focus on upsetting thoughts, the deeper you sink into depression. In other words, your feelings will feed off of your thoughts. The worse you feel, the harder it becomes to focus on possibilities, rather than impossibilities.

After focusing on negative thoughts for a long period of time, you began to develop a negative attitude. Your attitude affects you, your surroundings and the occurrences or the situations that occur in your life. With a negative attitude, you began to attract more un-welcomed situations and circumstances. At that point, your thinking will get worse. You will feel down and out. By now your attitude is so bad that you are unable to recognize a positive situation or an opportunity if someone were to lay one on your lap! Your mind has become negatively slanted. Your mind is now "set" to seek and receive negative, undesirable situations. Like attracts like in the realm of your mind. In other words, you will get exactly what you are!

If you doubt this concept, I invite you to try a little experiment. Pick a day (preferably a day when you are off work or school), and intentionally look for things to get angry or upset about. Wake up that morning with the idea that you are going to actually look for negative situations. Look for and find negative things to get upset about in your home. Gripe at your family members. Allow your- self to become irritated at everything you can. Put a chip on your shoulder. If you should accidentally think of something enjoyable, quickly put it out of your mind. You actually *want* everything to be negative. By the end of the day, you will have created a mountain of negativity. You will feel badly, because all of your thoughts will be negative. You will notice that you will have a bad attitude. You will be miserable! If you did this for days, weeks or months, you would become depressed.

On the surface, this exercise may appear to be foolish. I first thought so too. But I desperately wanted to know why things in my life went the way they did. I could not gauge my emotions or temperament. I was out of control most of the time. I would allow other people to dictate my attitudes. So I tried this experiment. To my surprise, I noticed how everything started to snowball negatively. By the end of the day, I had learned a great deal about myself. Also, I had learned a lot about other people, and how I could affect them! Positive people simply stayed away from me. However, I did manage to attract other negative people to engage me in a "pity party" session! **We often go through life without stopping to figure out what is really going on. If you are in the habit of doing this, then I would bet that you are unaware of how much you affect others and vice versa.**

We humans are born with "psychic receptors", and are able to pick up "vibrations" from other people. We send and receive subconscious signals all the time. For instance, how many times have you been thinking about someone whom you have not seen in a long while; only to run into or hear from them within the next couple of days? Most people mistakenly write off this natural function as coincidental or "chance." No matter how many times they experience it, they still falsely view it as an accident. **EVERYTHING IN LIFE HAPPENS FOR A REASON!**

I live miles from my mother, yet, she always knows ahead of time when I am having an unusual day or event. She may not know the particulars, but she does pick up enough of my "vibrations" to get a hold of me by telephone and find out what is happening. These are not unnatural "phenomenon." In fact, our ancestors in ancient Africa could carry on dialogues between villages as if they were standing right next to each other. Sounds strange, or unbelievable? Well, if you could talk to them now, they would think you were "strange" for not having this ability! **Our society has become so "high tech" that we have abandoned the most**

sophisticated technology ever known to humans ... OUR BRAINS!

So try this experiment and find out what kind of vibrations you are sending and receiving. You may find some of the reasons be- hind your bouts of anger or depression. The first step in dealing with your mind is to find out how it works or what makes it tick. Now after the first day of the experiment, it is critical that you get yourself out of this negative state of mind before you go to bed. How do you do so? Simple! You just reverse the process in your mind.

Get out a sheet of paper and make a list of positive things or situations that make you happy. List all the good things about your life. Are you healthy? Do you have a roof over your head to protect you from the cold nights? Do you have a family or friends? The list could be one or more pages. **YOU MUST BEGIN TO APRECIATE WHAT YOU HAVE NOW IN ORDER TO GET YOURSELF IN THE FRAME OF MIND TO REACH FOR MORE!**

Next, sit up straight. Take ten deep breaths. Breathe slowly. Inhale through your nose and slowly exhale out of your mouth. As you inhale, do so to the count of ten. Next, hold your breath for an- other count of ten. Then exhale to the count of ten. Again, breathe deeply through the nose to the count of ten — hold your breath to the count of ten — exhale to the count of ten. Repeat this process at least six times. After you have finished the breathing exercise, just lie back and relax with your eyes closed. Turn all of your thoughts inwardly. Forget about all of your cares or concerns, and just ... R-E-L-A-X.

You must use your imagination when you deep-breathe. As you inhale, imagine the air is coming into your body in the form of your favorite color. *(Many people think of light or sky blue as a peaceful color. I use black, as it represents absolute calmness to me.)* Also, think about the positive things that you listed. Think about things that make you feel great! Crowd your mind with thoughts that make you feel fortunate to be alive! Relive happy experiences. Everyone has had happy experiences. RELIVE THEM! Use them to get yourself in a positive frame of mind. When you think good, you feel good! As you exhale, do so to the color of your least favorite hue. This symbolizes your resolve to purge your mind of negative and crippling thoughts. You are exhaling negativism from your existence. So you are bringing in (or inhaling) positive thoughts and releasing (or exhaling) negative thoughts! This process is just as important to our existence as any other.

After you feel better, your mood will be lighter. Next, go to your family and explain to them why you were in such a "funky" mood all day. Apologize to them. Now that you are in a great mood, the whole day will be remembered as humorous. You can share your experience with them. You will all have had a very valuable experience. You will have first hand knowledge about the rules of cause and effect! You will know that bad thinking can only make a bad situation worse!

The next day, continue the experiment. Only this time your aim is to think only positive thoughts. When you wake up, go over the list of positives that you made the night before. Repeat the deep breathing exercise. Then add more positive thoughts to your list that you may think of. Keep the list with you throughout the day. Anytime you get a positive or refreshing thought, add it to the list.

Spend the entire day actually looking for positive situations. Take the time to express positive things to your family members and friends. If someone tries to dump their negative thoughts on you, quickly reverse the situation by finding positive things to tell them about themselves. Decide to let nothing negative linger in your mind. Whenever negativism creeps in, do the breathing exercise again. Then look over your list of positives. Pretend that you are the president of your own company and each thought that enters your mind are guests coming to visit with you. If the thoughts are positive, let them in and entertain them; do business with them. If the thoughts are negative, have your executive secretary make them wait in the hallway or ask them to leave. Today, you only have time for positive thoughts or guests!

Throughout the course of the day, you will notice that you simply feel great! You will have a terrific attitude! Try this second half of the experiment (the positive focusing and the breathing), everyday. The more you conduct this part of the experiment, the better

you will feel. If you get good at it, your whole life can change! What does that mean? It means you will always have a great attitude! If you have a great attitude, you will began to see things differently. You will be in the position (mentally) to see opportunities that you could only have seen with the right frame of mind! *(Note: If you just can't seem to shake your depression, you may need to contact a professional therapist for further evaluation. Try to find one that believes in natural, wholesome remedies.)*

Now that you have a proper attitude, you are prepared to move ahead in life. You must channel your new attitude in a certain or definite direction. You must have goals. Your life long goals are simply your "big picture." They are your pull toward the future. The most important thing about having goals is that they give you something to shoot for. Again, it is like taking a trip. If your goal is to drive from New York to California, you will remain "fixed" on that goal until you arrive. What if you have a flat tire halfway there? Do you abandon your overall goal of driving to California? Of course not. You simply do what is necessary to get back on the road to your destination. (You change the flat tire.)

It is likewise with all of your goals in life. You must not let life's "flat tires" keep you from focusing on your goals.

Usually, there will be trying times before "arriving" at your destination. But if your attitude, faith and belief systems are in place, you will be fortified with everything needed to accomplish what you have your sights set on.

But first you must have goals. Without goals, you are ways getting blown around by the cross-currents of life. You will be like a tumbleweed on a cold, windy day; always moving, yet never really going anywhere in particular. Goals are directions and with the proper attitude, your goals will pull you towards them. Goal seeking with the proper attitude and purpose will definitely point you in the right direction — your chosen direction!

People who manage to reach their goals in life tend to behave pretty much in the same manner. They are basically the same type of people. The same holds true for people who do not set and reach goals.

Let us look at one very important difference: Successful, goal oriented, goal-reaching people are usually "sticklers for detail." They leave no stone unturned. They are committed to follow through on even the smallest detail. It does not matter how large or small the task might be. They put their signature of excellence on all of their endeavors.

If you asked John Johnson, the publisher of Ebony Magazine, to sweep streets, I could almost guarantee that he would be the best street sweeper on the block. He would not leave a stone unturned. He would sweep and re-sweep until every speck of dirt was swept away! He would check his work again and again until he was sure to have met with perfection. The average person would merely sweep once and then say, "I don't have to go over that street again. I already swept it. Besides, it can't be that much dirt left… it doesn't matter!" I call these people, "It don't matter people." It is virtually impossible for these people to produce meaningful, long lasting successes in their lives because there are too many instances in their lives when things just "don't matter."

The alarm clock goes off, but they sleep another ten minutes be- cause "it don't matter." They fail to eat a healthy breakfast because "it don't matter." When they arrive to work or school, they "chill" or goof off for the first 15 to 30 minutes because "it don't matter." At lunch, they will throw away valuable time that they could have devoted to studying for that exam or finishing an important project because "it don't matter." At the end of the day, they leave a small portion of their work undone, "I'll get that little bit tomorrow, it don't matter", they tell themselves.

These people fail to realize that all those small "it don't matters" add up. They are forever behind, or late, or waiting on "someday." Secondly, and more important is the fact that they are establishing a mindset that makes it harder to follow through on the really big matters! Unless you are use to taking care of the little matters, you will not even recognize the big matters! Big matters are made up of a lot of little matters. I have seen marriages end because of a hundred little "it don't matters."

Many of our youth have turned to drugs and gangs because they think they just "don't matter." All too many brothers and sisters are cursing their blackness, and yet refuse to study their African history because they mistakenly believe that their roots "don't matter." **EVERYTHING MATTERS!** Fortunately, there is a simple way to change your life from don't matter to do matter! It may not be easy at first, but it is so very simple. The first thing to do is to decide that everything matters! Even if it does not appear to be so.

Start some simple exercises. At night when you get out of those dirty clothes, place them in the hamper, or hang that suit jacket up as soon as you take it off, rather than throwing it over a chair "for now." Make sure you spend some time each evening with your family members. Decide that it matters how their day went. Clear the table after supper — get those dishes done now not later. If you are a student doing your homework, decide to read a little extra, go the extra mile. If you brought extra work from your job, skip the Ellis Show and get it done, Tracee will understand. Ideally, you should make sure that all of today's work is completed before leaving work. Start tomorrow off on the right foot! During break time, take your break only if you have earned it. But, if that little voice in the back of your head says "work," then you stay and work. (That little voice is always right!) When the clock alarm rings in the morning, forget that snooze, get up immediately. That snooze button will set a precedent for the whole day… snoozers lose! Get up! Spend that valuable ten minutes in quiet reflection or in prayer. It will set the tone for the entire day.

You must determine that every project does matter no matter how small or insignificant it may appear. If you are vacuuming, move that couch and clean under there too. Not only because it is filthy under there, but realize that this simple action reaffirms that you fully understand everything matters!

Try this exercise for 30 days. You will be amazed at how your life can change. You will be an action person. You will find out just how much all those "don't matters," do matter! When you get good at handling all of the small matters in your life, you will be ready to set and start achieving your goals. You will definitely be heading in a direction that matters!

Once, I was talking with a group of young Brothers and Sisters about life in general, and specifically about some of the pitfalls that Blacks stumble upon and wallow in from time to time. Of- ten, we let negative racial impressions go unchecked. There are too many psychologically damaging games that we play that actually reeks havoc upon us… generation after generation. Too many seemingly unimportant things that we think "don't matter" that prevents us from achieving mental wellness and inner happiness.

For instance, we call ourselves nigga because "it really don't matter." We seek to look like other races by straightening our hair and bleaching our skin, "cause it don't really matter." We neglect to learn any of our African History… because after all, "that stuff don't really matter!" True enough, each of these things by them- selves probably "don't matter." But the accumulation of them all sums up to really, really B-I-G MATTERS!!

If we made it a goal to get rid of these put downs, one by one, we would soon find that the pain of being African is by and large, self-inflicted! People, we simply must change if we are to move on from where we are now. Individually and collectively, we can change… yes we can attend to all of the seemingly small matters and indeed grow and develop into the bold and proud people we once were; once upon a time. Give your life direction. After all, it is your life! Come to know that you were placed on this earth for a reason. Each and every human born in this orb known as earth can be of value to humankind. KNOW THIS TO BE TRUE!

Direct your present — Direct your future— Direct your life!

11

UNSHACKLED

Shackled minds are trapped in the lowly sphere of confusion, mis- understanding and corruption. They spend a lifetime without ever coming to the realization that they are bound to every fiber, every membrane and every cell that makes up what we call earth. We are in this thing together. Come to know this, and your stay in this realm will be a joyous journey. **Rare is the genius who comes to the understanding that all of humanity are but pieces of the same cosmic and global puzzle.**

You must understand and accept the fact that *you* can control your world with your "**thinking**." You do not use drugs to run from your challenges in life. You do not use or accept alibis like "it's the White Man's fault." You go a step beyond average Blacks by making sure that you have a working understanding of the histories of your people! You know that our past anchors us to the present and ushers us into our future.

In your quest for excellence, leave no stone unturned. Educate yourself. Spend time in the library. Go to the bookstores. Go to school. Give your life direction. Then diligently work to free your mind... stand tall; look neither to the right nor the left, but focus straight ahead. You are the one who has been so destined to hold the keys to your mind shackles; **your mind, your shackles, your power and ultimately... your choice**. FREE YOUR MIND!

-THE END-

I PUSH ON

*WHEN THE HEAVY WEIGHT OF OPPRESSION
DOWN UPON MY SHOULDERS . . .
I REJOICE, BECAUSE THOSE SHOULDERS
ARE MADE STRONGER,
AND I PUSH ON —*

*WHEN THE WINDS OF "MINORITYSHIP" HOWL
IN MY EAR. . .I REJOICE BECAUSE RARITY
IS A VIRTUE,
AND I PUSH ON —*

*WHEN MY OWN KIND WHISTLE WITH ENVY
AS I CLIMB LIFE'S LADDER . . . I REJOICE FOR
I CAN SEIZE THE OPPORTUNITY TO LEAD,
AND I PUSH ON —*

*WHEN CONFUSION AND MISUNDERSTANDING
CRAM THEMSELVES INTO MY MIND . . . I
REJOICE FOR YET ANOTHER OPPORTUNITY TO
LEARN AND PLACE ANOTHER FEATHER OF
WISDOM IN MY CAP,
AND STILL I PUSH ON —*

WHEN DEPRESSION AND DESPAIR INVITE
THEMSELVES INTO MY PEACEFUL WORLD . . .
I REJOICE FOR THEY BRING LESSONS THAT I
MUST BE TAUGHT, AND CAST REFLECTIONS, OF
MY INNER BEING, AND I AM LEFT
EVEN MORE ENLIGHTENED!
AND I PUSH ON —

AND AS I PUSH ON, I AM COMFORTED
BY THE EVER-PRESENT
GOD ALMIGHTY . . .
AND I AM THUS CARRIED ON!

Almas J. Sami'

AFTERWORD

THE CHANGE BEFORE THE NAME

As I speak to various groups, the one topic that seems to occupy the thoughts of most people is my name, whether they be African Americans or people of other races. Where did I get such a "strange" name? And why have I chosen to follow the path that I have taken? Although I understand the nature of such questions, I am caused to wonder if they may not be the wrong questions or at the least, inappropriate probes. It is like questioning why a man has chosen to take the pebble from his shoe.

I am constantly told by Blacks that a name change would not *"make a difference."* All I can say to them is; 'take the pebble from your shoe and see for yourself if it makes a difference.' See if it makes a difference in the way in which you approach life. I could talk and write about the power-enhancing benefits until I am Black *and* blue in the face. However, one cannot truly comprehend my tirades without having experienced the might of reconnecting one- self to a grand past with names that goes beyond our existence as slaves. It is like trying to explain to someone the difference be- tween making love, and having sex. If one has yet to experience love, then he is apt to mistakenly believe that the two are one in the same. You could spend a life time trying to show them the tremendous distinction, yet they will not fully appreciate the contrast until they have met with love. I tell people to give it a "sample" or "trial run" and see for themselves. Give it a try for just six months. For six months introduce yourself with a name that is reflective of our heritage before slavery.

It will virtually change the way you presently view Blackness, and unfortunately, you will also learn to what extent most Blacks hate or attempt to disregard Blackness. You will quickly gain the respect of other races because you will represent your race in a proud and respectful manner. When you tell someone your name, you are in essence, giving them your background... you bring to bare a host of past experiences and histories of your people. Our history goes far beyond the few years of our comparatively insignificant existence in this country... I believe our names should reflect that fact!

It has been a few years now, since I first changed my names, {or to put it more accurately, since I *chose* my name}. The feelings I had upon leaving the courthouse, along with my wife, Kai *(West African name meaning lovable)*, will be forever stamped in my mind. I felt both relief and heaviness. Heavy of heart because I knew that I must face my father and other family members with the news. And relief because I had finally done what I had for years considered an imperative. As fate would have it, the first meal we ate afterwards was an African meal, prepared by a friend from Senegal, West Africa.

The act of actually going down to the courthouse and "*doing*" it took over 10 years. My first encounter with the concept came in the 60s. The ex-heavyweight champion, Muhammad Ali was on the evening news explaining to reporters why he chose to rid him- self of his "*slave name.*" I loved and admired him as Cassius Clay, but even as a seven year old boy, I felt something special when this great boxer became a great man. Years later, when Kareem Abdul-Jabbar changed his name, I felt a special kinship to him. Some- how, he seemed to have more pride and internal strength than most men that I saw on my television. He was, in my opinion, a thinking man. At any rate, I felt as if I were missing out on some- thing very special.

My brother, Mustafa chose his name after becoming a Muslim in 1978. I was so proud of him! This act, as far as I was concerned, separated him from the pack. He joined the ranks of people I most admired. Yet, I could not muster the courage to follow suit. Occasionally, I would ponder and agonize over the prospects, why, I even went as far as to pick a name that I thought reflected who I am. Somehow, I would always end up placing it on the back burner. Then, in 1987, three separate occurrences made it impossible for me to continue living with an *imitation* name, and toting the bag- gage that comes with a *pseudo* designation that most African Americans consider "*Christian*" names.

The first incident involved me and another brother while attend- ing a political gathering. We all had on name badges. My friend who happened to have the same last name as one of the White members mentioned to the young White man that they may be distant relatives, in view of their common surname. The White fellow was obviously embarrassed as he felt the eyes and ears of the other Whites upon him. His embarrassment quickly turned into anger, and he coldly reminded my buddy that slaves took the names of their "former masters." I saw a look on my friends face that I had never seen before. A look that words can hardly explain. His pain, (and mine) was obvious though. It was if we were trying to snuggle up to everyone in that room. "*See boss, I'm jess like you suh… maybe we is even kinfolk*!"

At that moment, I did not realize I would feel that same trepidation only a few months later. As the owner of a small painting company, I had just completed a job for a White client whose name was the same as mine, which was Stevenson. After inspect- ing my work he said, ' I'm very pleased with the job. You do good work.' I beamed with pride and retorted, 'Of course I do good work, I'm a Stevenson!' No sooner had those words rolled off my lips, did I feel an indescribable frailty. We peered into each other's eyes for a brisk second that seemed like an hour. In fact, there was not a word that passed between us, yet that fleeting moment was filled with a history that spanned the entire 120 plus years since the end of slavery. I came to realize that no matter how much I had thought that name belonged to me, it was not mine! My people had not come about that name by way of pride or dignity. That slave name, like so many other bitter vestiges of that era came as the result of a people in search of acceptance. It came to me in the same tradition of the conked hair styles, the bleaching creams, and the total disrespect and disregard of Blackness! I did not then, nor do I now feel ashamed of the legacy of slavery. However, I did quickly come to the realization that I could do something that our fore parents could not do, and that was to reach back and make things as they "s*hould*" have been.

Ideally, at the time of the emancipation of our people, they "*should*" have had the mindset to claim their names, or at least names that reflected their heritage prior to coming to this land. But how could they? Blacks were thoroughly sold on the notion that they were inherently inferior. They had been arduously taught for centuries that "**Africaness**" (meaning anything of or from the Motherland) was less than whole, less than human, and less than White. They were sold a bill of goods that left them actually feeling inferior to Whites, resulting in a consuming hatred of themselves. So they had no choice but to grab a hold of something. And since White supremacy had been entrenched so deep within their psyches, it was only natural for them to cling on to what was familiar to them ... and that was the names and ideals of their former masters or at the very least, a notable White male of the time. It had to be a name that supported the fabrication that White was superior. The inclination of an African name never even *occurred* to ex-slaves! It was simply easier for us to take an Anglo name because we wanted, indeed, cherished White acceptance.

It did not have to make sense or appeal to logic. As an example of the mindset at the time, I call your attention to the blockbuster book, "*ROOTS,*" written by the late Alex Haley. As you will recall, Kunta Kinte' had a daughter named Kizzy. Kizzy was later sold to a man named "masa" Lea. She subsequently had a son whom they called Chicken George Lea. Years later while George, now fully grown was away in England, his wife and sons were sold to a "masa" Murray, henceforth, their surnames became Murray.

Now here is the clincher. After the Civil War, Chicken George returns and eventually lived with his sons. Oddly, the sons did not change their last name back to that of Chicken George Lea's last name! They kept the surname of their more recent "masa" Murray! Apparently, it made no since whatsoever to take the name of their father. They had as much, if not more of a paternal relationship with their former "masa" as they did with their own natural father who lived with them!

I remember watching the "*ROOTS*" television mini-series. I agonized when "Fiddler" told Kunta, 'It don't make no never mind what a nigga's name is no how.' As the slaves stood and watched Kunta Kinte' being beaten to within an inch of his life, they could not comprehend why he was so adamant about keeping his rightful name. "Toby is yo name cos dats whut da masa dun tol you." That was an African Americans' outlook 122 year ago. Today's average African American is more likely to say something like "It doesn't really matter what your name is, the only thing that matters is what you are." We stand alone as the only people on earth who would even dream of uttering such a statement! Our people were confused then, and regrettably, we are still confused today!

These thoughts and many more like them raced through my mind during that brief micro-second in front of this White Stevenson's house. I knew this name could not have possibly meant to me what it meant to him. I felt as if I were an orphan child, clinging onto the leg of a potential parent… the name felt different. The label that I used to sign with pride was now a source of shame!

The third occurrence that closed the chapter on my slave name was a much more positive one. Shortly after the debacle with this White client, I decided to change my name on my business cards. I took my brothers' last name. It was a name that I had always liked, and respected. A name that sets our family on a new course, one that our off-spring will now carry with pride into the future. When examining our family tree, one can easily see that the buck stops with our generation.

We have broken a horrible bond and made all of our ancestors proud. (**Sami'** , pronounced "*Sahmee*", is very ancient. It is also pronounced **Samia,** an Eastern African Tribal name that goes back many years. You may also see

Samihi or ***Saami'*** In proper Arabic or Islamic it is spelled **Abdul-Sami.** And of course you will encounter the ancient Kemetian (Egyptian) name; **Sami Ra Maati,** which means **"Double Wisdom Double Truth".**)

Incredibly, many people today question why African Americans of- ten choose Arabic or Muslim names! It is simple. Most of the early Arabic people and Muslim's were Black. In fact, the people in the area of what is now referred to as the "Middle East" were Black for centuries before more Whites continued to spread throughout the area and intermarry with the predominantly Black population. Just as the so-called "Egyptian" population grew lighter with the passage of time. The further back you trace the regions origin, the blacker the populous becomes. Many mistakenly think that White Arabs are the only Arabs. Nothing could be farther from the truth. The same holds true for many of the early Hebrews. The really beautiful thing about our opportunity here in America is that we can take a continental approach to the Motherland. In other words we can draw from all corners of Africa and claim it as our own. Even though most of us came from West Africa, our perspective should be Pan-African! All of Africa is ours! If we would have had this approach 500 years ago, we never would have sold one another out and rendered ourselves slaves for others. So do not take a tribal approach to the choosing of your name or your ancestors land. Kenya belongs to you just as much as the Sudan, or Senegal, or Nigeria, or Ethiopia, etc. We are indeed unique in this regard — our scope is much larger. All of Alkebu-lan is our birthright!

I noted instantly, that I felt a pride that I had never comprehended. It is as trying to explain to someone what "bliss" feels like. Unless one has felt it for themselves, they would have no basis for completely understanding the feeling.

The name *"took"* me! As the days went by, it became harder and harder to think of myself as a Stevenson. The name was simply no longer good enough for me.

No, I did not feel a hatred towards Whites. In fact, I felt less hostility towards them. The anger and resentment left me. I now realize that my hatred for them was a mere reflection of jealousy and deeply rooted envy. Most of us feel it, but few of us will explore our minds far enough to come to grips with our inner most feelings and thoughts... our fears! We are surface dwellers; afraid to delve into the deepest darkest recesses of our minds.

{This is most unfortunate, because the deep, dark passages of our minds are the only places that truth for us is revealed! Other races may choose to perceive darkness as less than desirable and evil, but for us, darkness has to mean enlightenment and yes, GODLY! The more darkness we invite into our world, the closer we get to truth, happiness and whole- ness! We must redefine darkness!}

My bliss even took me beyond the one major obstacle that always haunted me. It was the realization that I would surely hurt my father by rejecting his last name. How could I explain to him that I was rejecting the name and only the name? How could I make him know that I loved him infinitely, even though I could no longer carry the name he called his? How would he face his friends and our relatives? Would he reject me, as surely as I was rejecting the Stevenson name? I had to come to grips with these questions. But no matter what, I could not go back to that shame-riddled name! I am not a slave, thus the name had become moot as far as I was concerned.

The thing that helped me was the knowledge that our great ancestors believed that we are watched by those loved ones who came before us. As I believed this to be true, I began to think of how proud they are of me now that they have witnessed what I have done. Even though I do not know their actual names, I do know for a fact that they can identify with Sami' much more than they can Stevenson!

I am also comforted by the pride on the faces of brothers from Africa when they learn that I have changed my name. Many of them wonder why more African Americans do not follow suit. Surprisingly, there have been many White Americans who have asked the same question. In fact, upon learning that I had change my name, a fellow (a self-professed klansman no less), called me and said, "congratulations" and with that, he politely hung up the phone. He may not have like me, but he had no choice but to respect me. On the other hand, I have witnessed some Whites who, in a sick, psychotic sort of way, felt as though I were person- ally rejecting them by ridding myself of that unwanted baggage! I pity them.

The name change lends a kind of dignity that few Blacks in America can identify with. I know I could not fathom such a pride before I made the change. The greatest thing is to share that warm feeling with other African Americans who have also chosen their names. It is a brotherhood and sisterhood that is truly fantastic!

My children have an understanding I wish I would have had at their ages. As they study African History, I think of how much more inspiring it would be if the great African Americans that came before them would have had "*proper*" names! African names would make the Black greats instantly distinguishable or more readily recognizable in libraries and bookstores. **(This is a very important distinction since most public schools will not readily make that distinction for our children; for instance who would tell our children that the great Greek sage Aesop was actually an Ethiopian who lived in Greece?)**

Each generation has brought us closer to a 180 degree turn from where we were a hundred years ago. It is my belief that the act of recapturing names should be a major aim of African Americans under 40 years of age. It would be a giant step toward becoming whole. Every generation should do something to bring us closer to the way things should be. We who are under 40 years of age have yet to make our mark. We have yet to do something significant that the next generation can build upon. I believe massive, collective name changes would lend a golden legacy down to our future generations. That most young African Americans still give pseudo, slave names to their sons and daughters is an unfortunate reflection of the depth of the mind shackling process that took place centuries ago!The battles fought during the 1860s removed the shackles from our hands and legs. The struggles of the 1960s took the wicked weight of the Jim Crow system off our necks. Now we must utilize our resources and precious time rediscovering our humanity.

It is interesting that most Blacks will tell me that names are unimportant, yet I have encountered more hostility from Blacks than Whites! Usually people from other races will ask me about my name, and comment on it. Yet I honestly cannot remember but a few times when an African American actually inquired. Most notice it, but I will invariably get either no response or at the least, a frown. This leads me to believe that these notions have occupied the minds of many of us all. **Somewhere, in the deepest crevices of our minds, we wonder if this may not be something that must be addressed. But, we are yet locked into a mindset that often makes it difficult to distinguish fact from fiction; real or imaginary avenues.**

Some of us are so confused that we mistakenly believe others will see us as fakes if we underwent a name change! Imagine that! Our world, indeed our existence is so upside down that we feel more at ease wearing a European name than an African name! I remember feeling the same way when

I first wore an African shirt back in the 1970s. I thought others laugh at me for trying to be something that I was not. However, I could sport my European duds around and feel totally "at home." There can also be a parallel drawn between Blacks' response to my name and our lack of a sensible reflex to Africans in general. A brother from Senegal once told me he discovered that Whites are more apt to question him about the motherland. Whites are curious about African governments, modes of thought and ways of life. Yet the average Black man would not show the slightest bit of interest beyond "what is it like to go to bed with African Women?!"

This odd behavior reflects the degree to which we will steadfastly refuse to look at ourselves! It also speaks volumes about how little respect we have for our women. There is much work to be done! Again, I reserve my criticism for my generation, not preceding generations.

I believe it is futile to condemn earlier generations for not under- standing or being unwilling to grasp new ideas. It is natural for the status quo to reject new thoughts and approaches to our ongoing concerns. If one would study our history in this country, one would notice that the same pattern has developed virtually every time we have made gains.

For instance, most slaves thought Harriet Tubman was insane for believing that Blacks should escape to freedom! Many of the older generation thought she was asking for too much... going too far. They had learned to live within the boundaries of familiarity. Again, when Booker T. Washington said we needed education, the older Blacks rejected him and said that education was useless. Later, the establishment Blacks lambasted Carter G. Woodson when he declared that we should set aside one week each year to study Black History. The many "miseducated" Blacks condemned him and said he would wipe away gains already made if he continued with the notion that Whites would accept as fact that Blacks actually had a history.

And when W.E.B. Dubois and Marcus Garvey rose and said there is a need for African Americans to form organizations such as the NAACP and the Negro Improvement Association, they were deluged with criticism from the established Blacks who said the ideas were a waste of time, and would take away from our efforts to earn a living. Many said we would alienate ourselves from Whites who were sympathetic to our cause!

Once again, we see the same pattern emerge when in the late 1950s and 60s young brothers like Martin Luther King and Malik Shabazz defiantly rose to say that we should do away with Jim Crow systems, and we ought to seek independence. It was the status quo who said things are fine the way they are, and we should learn to work within the system. They felt it was not worth our while to try to do away with separate drinking fountains and eating establishments. They thought the younger generation was "barking up the wrong tree" with all this talk about self-reliance and independent thought. They believed that we must be fully integrated with White society because we would not be "allowed" to do anything on our own.

So it is with this history in mind that I reach out to those of us who are young and eager for a new direction. Yes, I truly do believe that every 30 years or so, we rise and awaken to new possibilities and forge new avenues of thought, taking our race closer to a 360 degree turn-about from where we were 50 years ago, 100 years ago . . **.I submit that it is time that we reclaim our names! It is time that we began passing worthy names to our children, so that they may stand tall, and will be able to look every other race in the eye without the heavy baggage of carrying the bogus honor of former slave masters. Most young African Americans are proud of**

their Blackness. So, why shouldn't they have names that up- hold and further reflects that pride?

I am not at all suggesting that the older generations are not proud, strong people. I am simply saying that it is time to move on from where we are now. It is time for yet another change; to move closer to where our grand ancestors were who civilized the world. Nor am I admonishing our White brothers and sisters. I nevertheless submit that it is time we looked them in the eye as equals, for a change. At last we must come to the conclusion that we will never look anyone squarely in the eye until we are able to look into our own mirrors with a pride that resonates from within!

Oh yes, I am fully aware of the fact that there have been successful Blacks who bare White folks names. Many of them will be mentioned in a positive vein throughout this book. Understand that my prescription regarding name changes is designed to raise us *collectively*. There always have been, and will continue to be pockets of successful Africans. However, if we seek to deal with obvious Black self-hatred — if we are serious about solving Black on Black crime, and coming to grips with why we just can't seem to get our stuff together, then we need to take a step back and consider my proposition.

I am convinced that within our minds and hearts the majority of Blacks concur with my assessment of our condition. Deep within the minds of most of us, it is agreed that it is a shame for us to continue holding on to the baggage that we brought forth from slavery. But we are afraid that Whites simply will not accept us if we "*offend* them with *unusual* names." We are afraid that we will not be able to secure good jobs . We shutter to think of the abuse our children will suffer as a result of having "*strange*" names. But the worst truth to bare has to be that we simply do not believe that *rightful* names are *worthy* names.

In our hearts, we wished we could muster the courage to face the world as bold human beings on *our* terms, but we have deeply rooted and ingrained fears. As a result, we simply attempt to sneak through life, hoping and wishing that no one will notice our black- ness! Continually telling ourselves that it just would not make a difference or it is "*not really that important.*" I say it is indeed time to be fearless! For years, we have had *individuals* stand and push us ahead. But we have yet to make a *collective* rise.

Names... powerful names, courageous names, truthful names — *our* names, would give us a spring board for unity that we have never enjoyed since our arrival in this land! Who among us will deny the cold hard reality that disunity has been our most formidable enemy? Indeed, our enemy of enemies! Change it brothers; change it sisters... you will be absolutely amazed at the power of liberation! In fact, you will kick yourself for not having the courage to do it before! It is like a grand medicine that may have bitter qualities, yet in the long run, you will discover that its magnificent healing properties leave you stronger, more refreshed and more alive than ever before.

But like any medicine, you must adhere to the instructions or directions. Changing your name alone will not liberate your mind, for your mind should be liberated *before* the choosing of a proper name. Never change it in an attempt to *show* White people that you have arrived, as you should have nothing to *prove* to them!

In fact, your name should reflect your own inner growth and personality. Also, you must do it with your enslaved ancestors in mind. They did not easily arrive at a slave masters name. The process of taking other peoples names was laced with unspeakable, even un- imaginable horrors... so you are actually *paying tribute* to them by cutting the cord that continually links us to former owners.

I am often asked for guidelines for changing and choosing a proper name. It is critically important that you take the time to research and become familiar with your ancestors' arrangements and methods. **Never choose a name because it "sounds cool" or looks good on paper. Those reasons would merely reflect your lack of under- standing! Your name should be authentic in meaning and should ultimately be an affirmation or description of who you are, or what you should consciously strive to become! Every time you hear your name, it should plant a conscious or sub-conscious seed of direction! Your name should propel you like a sling shot through life with great momentum!**

There are many noteworthy books on the market that you should study. Among them are; **The Book of African Names by Chief Osuntoki, Golden Names for an African People-African & Arabic Names by Nia Damali,** and then there is the all encompassing book, **African Names-The Ancient Egyptian Keys to Unlocking Your Power & Destiny by Hehi Metu Ra Enkamit.**

Yes, I did manage to make the change. I did manage to explain to my father, and was able to show him that I still had a deep and inspiring love for him. I understand why he kept his name. I am proud of him and his generation. They struggled and sacrificed to bring us from the back of the bus to where we are today. I also know that both of my parents are proud of me. After all, they were the ones who taught me to go for what I deem to be the pursuit of truth. They taught me courage, and faith while always giving me boundless love. I return their love, yet I also have an eye for my ancestors who first arrived in this country; tired, cold, weary and uncertain of but one monumental significance; their magnificent and most RIGHTEOUS NAMES!

THE COURAGE TO BE ME

GOD GRANT ME NOT GOLD, NOR GLAMOUR,
NOR THE PRETTY, BUT WATCH OVER ME AS I
ASSEMBLE THE **COURAGE** *TO THINK THE*
RIGHT THOUGHTS; **COURAGE** *TO REST UPON*
MY CONVICTIONS ONLY; **COURAGE**
TO OVERPOWER MY FEARS; **COURAGE** *TO BE*
STRONGER THAN MY WEAKNESSES; **COURAGE**
TO RISE AFTER A FALL; **COURAGE** *TO STAND*
ALONE FORTHE SAKE OF RIGHTEOUSNESS;
COURAGE *TO SIMPLY DOTHE RIGHT THING*
AND SURELY. . .THE **COURAGE** *TO BE ME. I WILL*
DO THE REST IN SERVICE OF
YOU AND YOURS.

Almas J. Sami'

TESTIMONIALS FOR THE UNSHACKLED MIND LECTURE & BOOK SERIES

"With great sensitivity and understanding, he teaches in this book that we must empower ourselves to be in charge of our thoughts… If you have never been exposed to our history prior to the landing of the slave ships, you will be enlightened." **—Kathy Clay-Little, Publisher, African American Reflections Newspaper**

"Thank you so much for allowing me to enrich my mind with such positivity. Of course I'm referring to your book. I took it everywhere with me, and I have it highlighted throughout its entirety… again, thank you for writing such a powerful and positive book that has obviously touched me. I will definitely spread the word!"

—T.B. Warren, College Graduate

"'The Unshackled Mind' is about personal reflections and common sense. It is intended as a contemporary primer—a down to basic, thought provoking thesis designed not only to inform, but to uplift. Significantly, the message in 'The Unshackled Mind' is not targeted to academicians alone. 'The Unshackled Mind' is both an easily digestible and highly readable text, in which the author does not insist that the reader agree totally with his conclusions, but demands that they be given serious consideration." **—Dr. Runoko Rashidi, African Research Specialist**

"The gift is not the book, but rather the message that breaks through the social hypnosis that African-Americans are in." **—Keith "Smokey" Johnson, TV Show Host**

"Powerfully effective, astonishingly clear, a self-help book that will open your mind. Unshackled Mind is a clean, crisp look into the natural order of thinking... Read this book and discover the miracle that awaits you!" **—Michael Fergins, Realtor**

"This book is second in line on the 'must read' category — right behind Dr. Carter G. Woodson's 'Mis-Education of the Negro!'" **—Basil Kamau Atum, Educator**

"The original thought or purpose of any good book, is to cause the reader to THINK; I believe you will do just that. The words on these pages are well thought out!" **—G. Naji, High School Principal**

TESTIMONIALS FOR THE UNSHACKLED MIND LECTURE & BOOK SERIES

"I am pleased to say that I have met this man in real life and are one of the first people to learn from his wisdom of life about being an African American, and growing up around the hood. Almas' enlightening understanding inspired me during my very early 20s to make positive leaps in forward thinking about myself, the life of all African Americans, and how to psychosocially survive in a harsh and industrialized society." —**Rah Ethereal, Student**

"This work represents a fresh new approach to African Diaspora mind set…A triumphant gallop through your mind that connects our grand ancient past to our bright future, and shows the reader how to turn distant dreams into contemporary realities. It affirms that we are indeed headed back to greatness!" —**Dennis J. Smith, Automation/ Robotics Specialist**

"When I read the Unshackled Mind, I knew I was tapping into the mind and knowledge of a person that has been there. Experience is the best teacher. I highly recommend this Book." —**Prince Eromosele Aligbe, CEO, Out of Africa, Inc.**

"Your book offers inspiration, courage and direction to all people of all ages who want to be the best that they can be, in a world that is often lacking in reaffirmation. This is especially important for our children of African-American descent whose success will 'make this world a better place.'" **—Dr. Joseph & Aaronetta Pierce**

"Thank you for your letter addressed to President Mandela. Your book and your letter will be forwarded to President Mandela in South Africa. I read a few pages from your book and I think it is wonderful. It is a book that Black South Africans should read as well." **—Phakamile Gongo, Public Affairs, Embassy of South Africa**

"Great book. Thought provoking. I am honored to be an owner of your book. Thanks for sharing with the rest of us your insightful and motivational skills. I am looking forward to your lecture series." **—William R. Harris, MD Psychiatrist**

"A must read for those who work as change agents, and are in the Social Services arena." **—Charles Middleton, Organizer**

TESTIMONIALS FOR THE UNSHACKLED MIND LECTURE & BOOK SERIES

"Mr. Almas Jamil Sami' is on my reference and resource list as one of the most powerful speakers that I have had the opportunity to hear. When looking for words to describe him, the first that come to mind are forthright and straightforward. He is serious, with a sense of humor, sensational, motivational, and inspirational. I found that each of his messages had application to life as it really is. His steadfast professionalism is admirable. His book should be read by all and his speeches should be heard by all—young and old, Black and White." —**Ernest Spikes,**

Jr., President Texas Association of Black Personnel in Higher Education San Antonio Chapter And Chairman Education Committee, NAACP San Antonio Branch, Coordinator of Counseling St. Philips's College

"To assist in finding solutions to problems, one must be able to communicate and define the situation and its parameters. Bro. Sami' serves in the capacity of a communicator. His lectures, his Television Hosting attributes, and his written words have allowed communication to begin and foster on two continents." **—Beverly Harris, School Teacher And Nias Harris, President, Harris Enterprises**

"Your presentation of 'The Unshackled Mind' was informative, inspirational and enlightening. I plan to continue to use your book as a source of empowerment and as a tool for teaching our students. Your presentation is one that should be heard by those constituents within and apart from education. The students ex- pressed to me that you were honest, full of wisdom and you captured their undivided attention. It was also obvious that you are dedicated to giving back to the community." **—Phyllis R. Thompson, Program Coordinator for Minority Affairs University of Texas * San Antonio**

"When I think of Almas Jamil Sami', I am reminded of an old Yoruba saying; 'Often what we are looking for is near us; it is only our lack of knowledge which prevents us from seeing it.' It is with this clear understanding of African Americans, and our lack of knowledge of ourselves as an ancient and historical people, that Almas Jamil Sami' is dedicated to change. He believes, and ex- plains in his 'Unshackled Mind Lectures,' that the answers to many of the problems that plague our communities, can be found not only within our own cultural experiences; but, with self-knowledge it can be illuminated within our own selves as well." **—Keith "Smokey" Johnson, Host of "The Umoja Circle"**

TESTIMONIALS FOR THE UNSHACKLED MIND LECTURE & BOOK SERIES

"This man, who in my eyes, after hearing him speak, represents African American men in a positive way. His speaking about his life (where he's been and how far he has come) is so inspirational and motivating to the point where you feel like you can get up from wherever you are in life and be the best at anything if you are determined and if you use your mind! Beyond that, he makes you feel proud to be an African American. I wish he could speak to all the little boys and girls across the world and spread his message because that's where it needs to start. Keep up the good work my brother, I love you for who you are and who you represent." **—Rita Thompson, Purchasing Agent, Alamo Workforce Development, Inc.**

"Almas Jamil Sami' is a powerful writer and lecturer who seeks to enlighten and uplift those with which he comes in contact. Sami' has many thoughts and opinions about what needs to be done to empower our communities. He has something to say and we should listen!" **—Traci Brooks, Public Speaker and Poet**

"This world is full of eloquent speakers; however, Bro. Sami' is one of a few who speaks with such commitment, passion, and conviction that you're unable to leave one of his sessions unchanged. He has a message of empowerment for all mankind." —**Vernon Cooper, CEO, Coski Enterprises, Inc.**

"Almas Jamil Sami' is like a breath of fresh air to the plight of African Americans. Unlike many of our other intellectuals, we spend too much time as in Bro. Sami's words having "pity parties." He places the responsibilities right where they rest . . . with us! He emphasizes one taking primary responsibility for their actions which will result in solutions. In order for African Americans to actually have freedom, they must learn how to think in terms of freedom. The ancestors are rejoicing that such a time has come for intellectuals like Bro. Sami' to pave the way for future Africans to take up their struggles with 'The Unshackled Mind.'" —**Bro. Alvin B. Hicks, Ancient African Research Specialist**

BIOGRAPHY

Almas J. Sami' (pronounced SAH-me) contributed 17 years of pain and failure into his powerful message. Born with ADD/ADHD, and a father by age sixteen, he went on to drug dependency, flunked out of two colleges, was homeless twice, filed bankruptcy, faced eviction four times, failed at over 70 jobs and businesses, suffered a complete nervous breakdown and later fought a two year battle against hepatitis and a crippling virus that attacked his immune system. His failures were the catalyst for his drive to study human nature and to learn why some people excel, while others fall short. Why some people live lives of fullness and passion while others merely exist or wallow at the bottom in seemingly every endeavor. His years of personal and historical study gives rise to his unique perspective on Black post and pre-slavery thought, i.e., why Blacks flourished magnificently in the ancient past and yet seem to languish on the bottom in modern times. Mr. Sami' recently utilized his understanding of thought/mindset deliberation and holistic medicine to overcome a lengthy and debilitating illness. Sami' went on to complete The Unshackled Mind, a book that opens the door to a NEW way to think and live for Blacks the world over. It is sure to cause rippling effects in the Black community for some time to come. Almas and is wife, Kai are now founders of Sohaja Publishing Company featuring Simba Lectures & Keynotes. His powerful lectures leave audiences feeling not only energized and empowered but actually establish new thinking patterns! He is currently a U.S. Air Force Disabled Veteran. Sami' has mentored troubled African American youth in alternative schools, detention centers and prisons throughout The United States. Born and raised in Clinton, Oklahoma, he now resides in Texas with his wife, Kai of over forty seven years They together have three offspring and five grandchildren. They have written three other books, **I Would Tell You These Things If I Were Your Father**, **Spirit, The Church Within US** and a children's book, **When Trees Could Walk**. Three CD's. Most of their CDs and speeches can be found on youtube.com under Almas Jamil Sami channel. They can be found on facebook.

BIBLIOGRAPHY

Karenga, Maulana. (2010) Introduction to Black Studies. Los Angeles, California: University of Sankore Press. This book compiles the latest material from a vast array of sources in the seven core areas of Black Studies: history, religion, sociology, politics, economics, creative production and psychology. He critically engages the most recent theories, research and developments in the discipline, bringing a fresh approach in response to new research and new interpretations within the Black Studies project.

Akbar, Na'im. (1984) Chains And Images of Psychological Slavery. Jersey City, New Jersey: New Mind Productions. In this book you will learn how to break the chains of your mental slavery.

Asante, Molefi Kete. (1990) Kemet, Afrocentricity, and Knowledge. Trenton, New Jersey: Africa World Press. A profound statement of the Afrocentric perspective.

Kunjufu, Jawanza. (1987) Lessons From History A Celebration in Blackness. Chicago, Illinois: African American Images. A Black history textbook that goes beyond "Negro" to African History, this book shows the strengths, weaknesses, victories, and mistakes of African Americans. Beautifully illustrated, it includes test questions and vocabulary exercises.

Kondo, Baba Zak A. (1988) A Crash Course In Black History: 150 Important Facts About Afrikan Peoples. Washington, DC: Nubia Press. African Facts.

Houston, Drusilla Dunjee. (1926) Wonderful Ethiopians of the Ancient *Cushite Empire.* Oklahoma City, Oklahoma: The Universal Publishing Company. Covers the Ancient Cushite Empire, Ethiopia, it's people, land and civilisation, prehistoric Egypt, the Paroahs, Arabian civilisation, Babylonia, Chaldea, Ancient India and Ancient Media and Persia among others.

Diop, Cheikh Anta. (1991) *Civilization or Barbarism. Chicago, Illinois: Chicago Review Press.* Challenging societal beliefs, this volume rethinks African and world history from an Afrocentric perspective.

Finch, Charles. (2000) *The African Background to Medical Science.* London, England: Karnak House Publishers. Essays in African History, Science and Civilizations.

ben-Jochannan, Yosef A.A. (1972) Black Man of the Nile. Baltimore, Maryland: Black Classic Press. Challenge and expose "Europeanized" African History. He points up the distortion after distortion made in the long record of African contributions to world civilization. Once exposed he attacks these distortions with a vengeance, providing a spellbinding corrective lesson in our history.

Blassingame, John W. (1973) The Slave Community. Oxford, England: Oxford University Press. Plantation life in the Antebellum South. It is one of the first historical studies of slavery in the US to be presented from the perspective of the enslaved.

Clarke, John Henrik. (2008) Article: Why Africana History? New York City, New York: Hunter College of the City University of New York. Originally published in The Black Collegian Magazine (1997). In the late 1960s through the late 1980s, the late John Henrik Clark was one of the foremost architects of the emerging discipline of Africana Studies/Africalogy as Professor of African World History in the Department of Black and Puerto Rican Studies at Hunter College of the City University of New York. He explored history's utility in moving an oppressed and subordinated people from a position of subjugation on multiple levels to full status as a self-sustaining, self-defining self-directed, free, and independent people on a global stage.

Amen, Nur Ankh. (1999) The Ankh: African Origin of Electro-magnetism. Brooklyn, New York: A&B Publishers Group. It behooves the African anthropologist to use every scientific discipline that modern technology has to offer, in the tradition of Chiekh Anta Diop,to acquire the correct perspective on African high culture and civilization. Now is the time for Africans to wrestle Egyptology from the clothes of the distorters of our civilization, by a more forceful and public attach on their lies. We must expose to the light of truth, every falsification and every clam of a European or

Woodson, Carter G. (1933) The Mis-Education of the Negro. Philadelphia, Pennsylvania :Oshun Publishing. "When you control a mans thinking you do not have to worry abut his actions." The thesis of Dr. Woodson's book is that African Americans of this day were being culturally indoctrinated, other than taught, in American schools. This conditioning, he claims, causes African Americans to become dependent and to seek out inferior places in the greater society of which they are a part. He challenges his readers to become autodidacts and to "do for themselves", regardless of what they were taught: History shows that it does not matter who is in power...those who have not learned to do for themselves and have to depend solely on others never obtain any more rights or privileges in the end than they did in the beginning.

Al-Mansour, Dr. Khalid Abdullah Tariq. (1992) San Francisco, California :First African Arabian Press. Welcome To Islam. Controversial Islamic leader Dr. Khalid Abdullah Tariq Al-Mansour offers a comprehensive look at Islam, the Muslim religion — its history, practices, literature, ambitions at proselytizing the word, and its role in the "New World Order."

Chief Osuntoki. (1970) The Book of African Names. Washington, DC : Drum and Spear Press. Chief Osuntoki explains the importance of ceremony surrounding the naming of a child. He explains proper birthright and how to seek the child's name. Lists of male and female names are also included and are categorized according to tribal regions of Africa.

Damali, Nia. (1986) Golden Names for an African People -African & Arabic Names. Grand Forks, North Dakota: Blackwood Press. Robbing peoples and countries of their rightful names was one of the cruel games that colonizers played on colonized people. Names are like magic markers in the long streams of racial memory, for racial memories are the rivers leading to the sea where the memory is stored. To rob people of their name is to set in motion a psychic disturbance that can, in turn, create a permanent crisis of identity.

Enkamit, Hehi Metu Ra. (1999) African Names-The Ancient Egyptian Keys to Unlocking Your Power & Destiny. Asian origin of Kemet and re-establish the link with our ancestors for the sake of our children.

CPSIA information can be obtained
at www.ICGtesting.com
Printed in the USA
FSHW021025040420
68808FS